# Dr Ali's
# Women's
# Health Bible

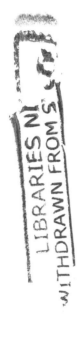
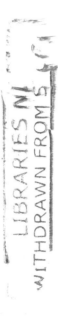

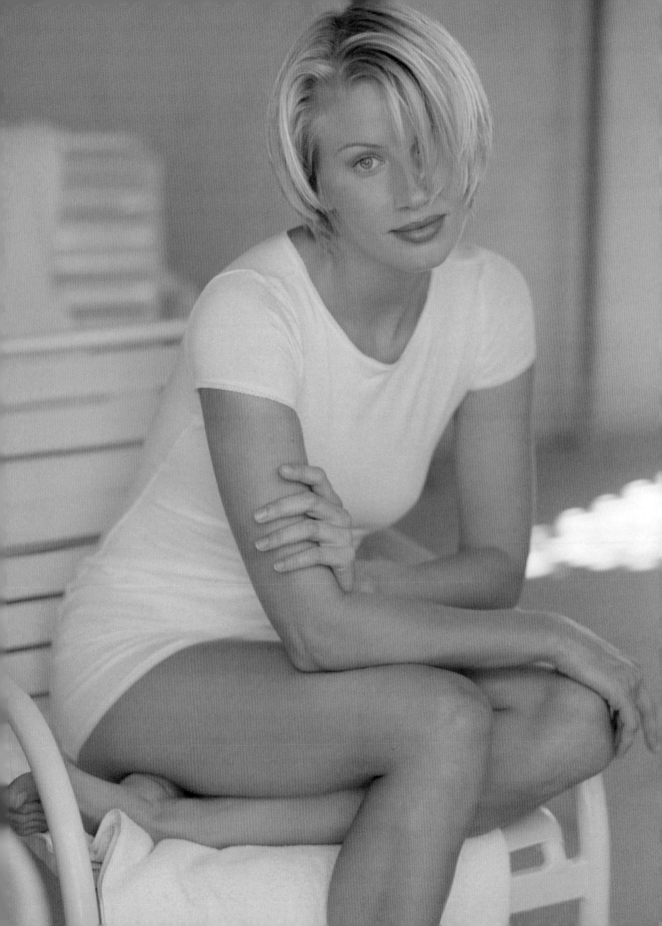

# Dr Ali's Women's Health Bible

## The essential guide to your health and well-being

# Dr Mosaraf Ali

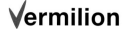

First published in Great Britain in 2006

1 3 5 7 9 10 8 6 4 2

Published by Ebury Publishing,
Random House,
20 Vauxhall Bridge Road,
London SW1V 2SA

Random House Australia (Pty) Limited
20 Alfred Street, Milsons Point, Sydney,
New South Wales 2061, Australia

Random House New Zealand Limited
18 Poland Road, Glenfield, Auckland 10, New Zealand

Random House South Africa (Pty) Limited
Endulini, 5A Jubilee Road, Parktown 2193, South Africa

The Random House Group Limited Reg. No. 954009

www.randomhouse.co.uk

A CIP catalogue for this book is available from the British Library

ISBN 0091902436
ISBN 9780091902438 (from January 2007)

All images © Getty, except on pages 55 and 160 © Alamy.

Illustrator: Bridget Bodoano
Designers: Isobel Gillan and Lawrence Morton
Editor: Caroline Ball
Copy Editor: Margaret Gilbey
Consultant Nutritionist: Fiona Hunter

**Disclaimer:** Although every effort has been made to ensure that the contents of this book are accurate, it must not be treated as a substitute for qualified medical advice.

   Always consult a qualified medical practitioner. Neither the author nor the publisher can be held responsible for any loss or claim arising out of the use or misuse of the suggestions made or the failure to take medical advice.

Printed and bound in Singapore by Tien Wah Press

# contents

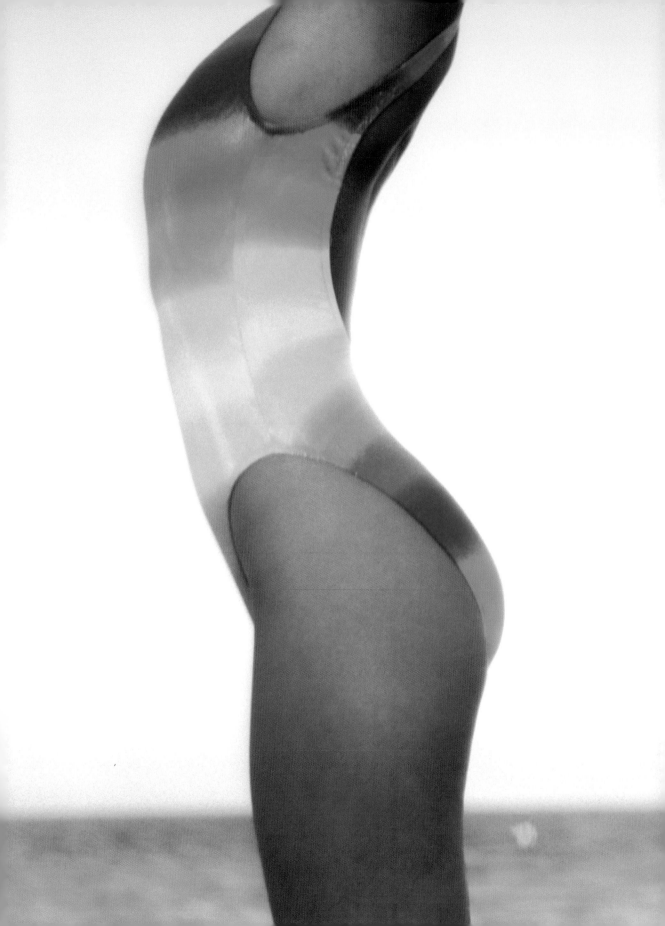

# introduction

When I opened my clinic in London in 1998, I soon found I was receiving many more women than men as patients – and the same is true today. Women have embraced complementary therapies more readily and, while not turning their backs on conventional medicine, recognize that a blend of the two, and a more holistic approach to health, provides more satisfactory answers to their problems and concerns.

This is exactly what integrated medicine does. After completing my medical studies, I specialized in complementary and traditional medicine, and have developed integrated medicine by drawing on a multiplicity of disciplines, taking whatever is best and most appropriate to the individual in any particular circumstance.

Many doctors nowadays rely on patients to tell them what the matter is. But when I see a patient for the first time I begin to assess her state of health from the moment she walks into the room. I note her posture and the way she walks, and her facial expression. I look at her skin (a poor or spotty complexion? flushed cheeks?) and her eyes (are they bulging or sunken? are there bags or dark shadows beneath them?) and for tell-tale signs such as thinning hair or a tightly held jaw. I listen not only to what she says but how she says it, whether her tone is confident or hesitant, high-pitched and excitable or flat and tired.

I will then ask her to stick out her tongue, perhaps feel her pulse (see page 90) and, if I feel it will be helpful, carry out iridological diagnosis to see what the irises of her eyes can tell me about her health. At this point, using my years of experience, I will have a fairly good idea about her general condition. It is then that I start asking relevant questions to confirm my assumptions, to form a firm diagnosis.

Often, by the time patients come to see me they have seen many other doctors and received previous diagnoses, which can sometimes be confusing, so I find making a fresh diagnosis is always useful. Moreover, I look into collateral issues such as digestion, sleep, stress, and aches and pains. Conditions such as constipation or panic attacks may not at first appear relevant to the original diagnosis, but they provide clues to a patient's general health and help me to make a more complete diagnosis, and so decide on the best form of treatment.

I came to write a regular column in a major British newspaper supplement because of its female readership. Family health still rests primarily in a woman's hands. Far more women than men care for the family's well-being: they prepare the food they eat, make appointments with doctors, nurse them through illnesses and read about health care.

In the first part of this book I take a look at why it is so important that a woman's health should not be considered and treated exactly the same as a man's. This means taking into account the less obvious ways in which women differ from men, ways that are not visible on the surface but which can make a big difference to the way women are affected by illness. One of the most frequently asked questions I get from my patients is: 'What type am I, Dr Ali?' There is a fascination with categorization of all sorts, from blood types to ancient ayurvedic classifications, and it seems that almost every woman patient I see is eager to know which she fits into. For this reason, I have included in **Part 1** some brief details that may be interesting in this respect.

**Part 2** is the core of my approach to health and well-being, expanding my basic Lifestyle Programme to emphasize relaxation and moderation, vital factors in maintaining a healthy balance. As well as practical examples of how the Lifestyle diet and exercise regime can be incorporated into a busy schedule, there is an MOT specifically tailored to women in different stages of life.

**Part 3** encompasses all aspects of women's health, from alleviating period pains or hot flushes to understanding anorexia, from the significance of a lump in the breast to enjoying a trouble-free pregnancy.

Through this book I hope that you will come to understand better how your body works in health and in ill-health, and that it will help you balance the physical, psychological and emotional aspects of your life. I also hope that it will prove an invaluable guide to whatever ailments, major or minor, you may have to face.

*Dr Mosaraf Ali*
*November 2005*

# why women need their own guide

Ideally, a woman's doctor should not only know about obstetrics and gynaecology, but also be trained in endocrinology, which deals with all hormonal functions, psychiatry, child care, skin care, weight management and nutrition as well as general health care. However, it is not uncommon for a gynaecologist to say glibly 'go and get some weight off' or 'get your stress sorted out', without being able to give complete guidance him- or herself. In this age of specialization, there are more specialists and fewer generalists. What every women needs is a generalist women's physician who understands women's specific problems and can deal with them – you simply cannot run a well-woman clinic without being able to deal with the whole range of issues faced by women in the course of their lives.

# part 1

At the moment, though, such facilities are astonishingly rare and so it is up to you to learn about how your own body functions, to recognize how it responds to different stresses and circumstances, and to know how best to treat it in the hope of being rewarded by a long and healthy life. A vital part of this is to understand something of the many ways in which women differ from men – differences that go far beyond body shape and the ability to have babies – and how very varied women themselves are, so that what may be right for your sister-in-law or your neighbour may not be right for you.

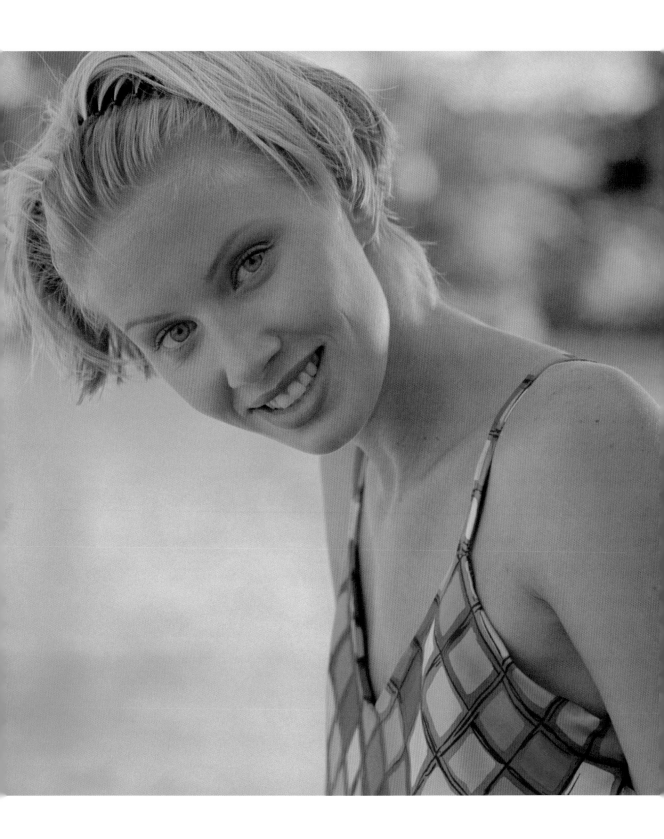

# chapter one

# women in the 21st century

Once, women's internal workings were considered a mystery and their minds unfathomable. Nowadays, all too often, the real differences between men and women are ignored or minimized. But equality doesn't mean sameness. Somehow, we have to reach a true equality that allows for a woman's feminine nature to be an integral part of her life and health care.

# Women's health & well-being Well-being goes beyond health. You can be technically healthy and yet not feel great.

Someone afflicted with, for example, migraine, menstrual cramps, chronic fatigue syndrome, general aches and pains, irritable bowel syndrome, frequent coughs and colds, insomnia, depression or panic attacks will probably show no, or very little, variation from the norm in physical health checks such as blood tests. Many women have perfectly normal periods and show no hormonal irregularities, yet they cannot conceive naturally. A medical examination can reveal so little of such suffering.

Although there are departments of gynaecology and obstetrics in hospitals and clinics to treat conditions that are specific to women, for most aspects of health men and women are generally treated in the same way and in the same place (economics plays a big role in this, and so does convenience).

Treating the disease rather than the person can be of particular disbenefit to women. To give just one example: steroids are commonly prescribed to sufferers of rheumatoid arthritis or MS. But men and women react to them very differently. A woman will find she gains weight and her face puffs up; she suffers from fluid retention and often has problems with her periods; she is likely to have trouble sleeping and have terrible mood swings or become aggressive. Men are much less likely to have any such troubling side-effects. Further problems that afflict women, such as excess body hair, hormonal weight gain, hair loss and PMS, are often misunderstood, misconstrued or dismissed as 'vanity matters'.

As women, you are routinely counselled not to take drugs or eat certain foods while you are pregnant, to safeguard the baby's health. But what about your own health? Artificial hormones, antibiotics, painkillers and other regularly prescribed drugs can have horrendous side-effects. Most of the hormones and fertility drugs have temporary benefits, but at a price. And drugs to treat endometriosis, for example, act by suppressing female hormones, thereby giving a boost to the male hormones all women also have, resulting in a gradual loss of femininity. Should you be subjected to drugs that tamper with your very being as a woman?

An additional, major contributor to women's ill-health is one that is mostly overlooked or underestimated: the stress brought on by the conflicting demands of modern life.

## A change in emphasis

It is my firm belief, based on years of experience, that the pattern and strains of modern life have altered the way a woman feels, looks and behaves. In traditional families women ran the affairs of the family and were called 'housewives' as they worked at home. The power they held was real and their pre-eminence in matters such as child-rearing, family health, domestic spending and, in wealthier homes, staff training and discipline was undisputed. However, in a money-based economy, wealth equals power and a healthy balance of duties and responsibilities can easily become distorted in favour of whoever holds the purse strings.

Suffragism, women's lib and equal rights appeared to do much to redress the balance of power, but in fact brought with them a new set of difficulties. Women discovered they had to work harder than their male counterparts to 'prove their equality'; some found they had to bury their femininity by mimicking a male style of

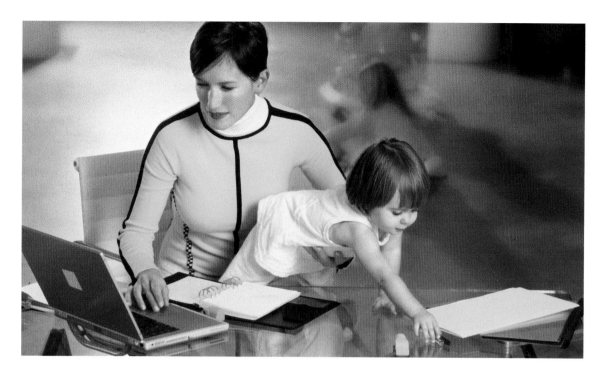

working or adopting a 'ladette' persona. Working women with a family often found the larger part of household chores and of maintaining the 'family glue' still fell to them, testing their energy levels to the limit; they would juggle job and family commitments and wrestle with guilt when one detracted from the other. Women who chose not to follow a career or paid employment found they lost status, and became defensive about their choice or guilty about not contributing to the family finances.

When body and psyche are put under strains like this, it obviously reflects on general health but also rebounds on women in perhaps an unfair way – on their womanhood itself. Stress hormones (such as adrenalin) are akin in nature to male hormones, and an increase in male-style hormones is one of the most unnatural things that can happen to a woman. Many conditions on the increase today – including polycystic ovary syndrome, infertility and some forms of obesity – stem from this shift in hormonal balance that stress induces.

## Listening to nature

A woman's body is perhaps more attuned to nature than a man's. One of the main reasons for this is that the effects of hormonal cycles are more prominent. It has frequently been noted that hormonal-based problems respond better to natural treatments than when tackled with strong medicines – fertility treatments with medicines often fail while natural ones (herbs, relaxation, diet) are more successful. Many couples, having given up trying for or having adopted a child, subsequently have their own, when the anxiety of not conceiving has gone. And heavy periods, menstrual cramps and pain, endometriosis, polycystic ovary syndrome, amenorrhoea and PMS, usually treated by hormones, often come back when the medicines are stopped.

# Sound advice from the past

Many newly qualified doctors still take the Hippocratic oath, by which they promise to take good care of their patients, not to harm, not to change them too much and to be compassionate. Unfortunately, few physicians today know much more about Hippocrates, the father of medicine, what he preached and why he was so important. Despite his demise nearly 2,500 years ago, much of what this Greek physician taught and practised has equal relevance today. Some of the main features of the preaching were:

- **We all have a healing power within us that keeps our body healthy and protects us through illness.** This innate power he called 'physis'. This is the root of words such as physiology, physiotherapy and physician itself, but the meaning has been lost because neither do physicians treat the physis nor is physiology about the knowledge of physis. Today's physicians do not believe in physis or natural/innate healing powers. The closest they come to accepting it is by talking about the immune system, which relates only to the means by which the body defends itself from external invasions of bacteria or allergens.

- **This physis or healing power can by itself cure about 80 per cent of illness, with medicines and other interventions required only for the remainder.** This is in direct contrast with much of modern medicine, where treatment or intervention is applied to most conditions.

- **Physis needs to be nurtured and kept active by simple means: good nutrition, massage, exercise and rest.** This makes sense – if you eat and exercise sensibly, rest enough and use massage to remove fatigue and improve circulation, you are likely to stay healthy, and if you do fall ill, such simple treatments will help to replenish lost energy and help the body to heal and recover quickly.

- **Hippocrates saw two opposing forces acting constantly within the body to maintain equilibrium or health.** Bacteria, hazardous pollutants and potentially harmful substances surround us and enter our bodies via injuries to the skin and mucous membrane through air, water and food. These form the pathogenic force ('pathos' = disease). Our body challenges them with the sanogenic force ('sanos' = health). When the sanogenic force suppresses the pathogenic force we remain healthy. If the pathogenic force overpowers our sanogenic force, then the result is disease or illness. When we are ill, we need energy to fight the illness – plus an additional boost to get back to optimum health. The best way to prevent and combat illness is to have strong sanogenetic reserves.

- **When the body is diseased or ill, any treatment should help the sanogenetic forces or healing power without ill effects.** Hippocrates was well aware of the dangers of aggressive treatment, and the modern version of his oath includes the promise: 'I will remember that there is art to medicine as well as science, and that warmth, sympathy and understanding may outweigh the surgeon's knife or the chemist's drug.'

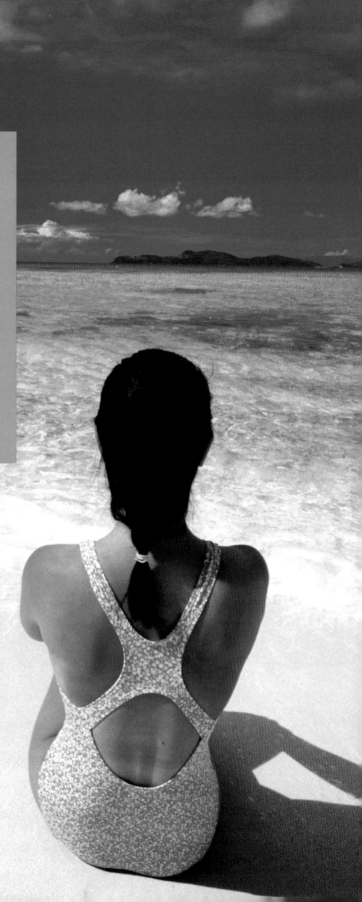

## CYCLICAL INFLUENCES

It is amazing how most natural phenomena are cyclical, and in fact the presence of cycles within our own body is a demonstration of how much we are a part of nature and open to being affected by cycles in the cosmos, the environment and the earth.

The sun (diurnal cycles within us), the moon (the monthly cycles of periods) and the planets (seasonal cycles) all influence our bodies. Our body clocks do not follow an exact 24-hour cycle but have to be reset each day by sunlight. And I have known several women whose ovulation or start of their periods always coincides with the full moon. Women living or working together long-term often have their periods more or less around the same time. This is partly due to a subconscious reaction to female pheromones, but it's also feasible that receptors in the brain are sensitive to these natural cycles.

*Galen, the great Greek physician-surgeon, and later Avicenna, the wise Persian physician, expanded this concept even further. They formulated six essentials for optimum health:*

**1 Food and drink** With a balanced, moderated diet our digestive systems function better. Sufficient nutrients provide the body with all its raw materials and other requirements, and they help the body fight off ailments. Herbs and spices have medicinal properties, while certain foods and beverages can damage the body if taken in excess.

**2 Air and environment** It is not pollutants in the atmosphere that alone cause ill-health. The temperature of the air, the pollen, viruses or airborne diseases, the smell of putrefying rubbish or sewers, and overcrowding of urban areas all affect the quality of the air. Low and high atmospheric pressure, storms and freak weather changes affect our well-being. Cold air causes mucus discharge and sinus problems.

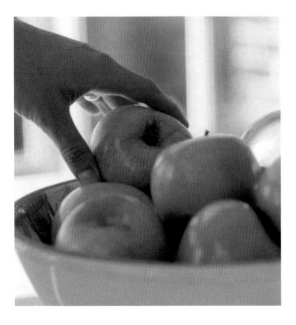

**3 Movement and rest** Anything done to excess can cause illness, especially if it is not mitigated by sufficient rest. Exercise and movement are beneficial, keeping the body strong and supple, but the energy consumed in physical activity takes time to be replenished. If overactivity becomes a habit and no time is given to the body to restore its energy then it gets run down.

**4 Sleep and wakefulness** Lack of sleep is a common cause of many psychological illnesses. A good night's sleep creates a positive mood and greater energy, and the body functions better.

**5 Eating and evacuation** Both eating too little and eating too much have serious health implications. People survive remarkably in times of famine, but nutritional deficiencies open them to infection and weaken their innate ability to regain a state of health. Poorly functioning bowels relate to numerous illnesses.

**6 Emotions** Emotional troubles manifest themselves in a mixture of psychological and physical symptoms, such as palpitations, anxiety and phobias. Depression brings on not only morbid thoughts and a poor sense of self-worth, but chronic fatigue, low blood pressure, poor concentration, lack of sleep, poor appetite and a slow pulse rate.

A woman's body is so sensitive to the influences identified by Galen and Avicenna that I would go so far as to say that following a lifestyle programme, such as I describe in Part 2, is almost essential. It may prove a tough discipline at first, but adopting it is a very important step, especially to overcoming hormonal and stress-related conditions.

# The differences between men and women

As I pick up the pen to write this, one thought comes straight to my mind – that this is a daring subject, practically taboo.

Most women in the developed world have been brought up, rightly, to see that they are the equal of men. But this has also led to a widespread, but wrong, belief, that they are the same as men. To suggest otherwise appears to condone labels such as the 'weaker sex' or 'fairer sex'. It is not considered politically correct to highlight ways in which men and women differ because this somehow undermines the equality women have so long fought for, and seems to indicate discrimination or favouring men over women.

Nothing could be further from the truth. Cleopatra and the Queen of Sheba were not the only women to have led armies of men into major wars, and history records numerous queens, female presidents and prime ministers. In the former Soviet Union, where I studied medicine, the entire medical force was dominated by women. Laws gave women special privileges. They had the same job opportunities and were paid equally, but they retired five years earlier than men. They took up tough jobs in the mines and in the road-building industry; they drove heavy-duty vehicles or trains, or flew military and commercial aircraft. Maternity leave could be extended to up to a year and a woman could retire after bearing her fifth child.

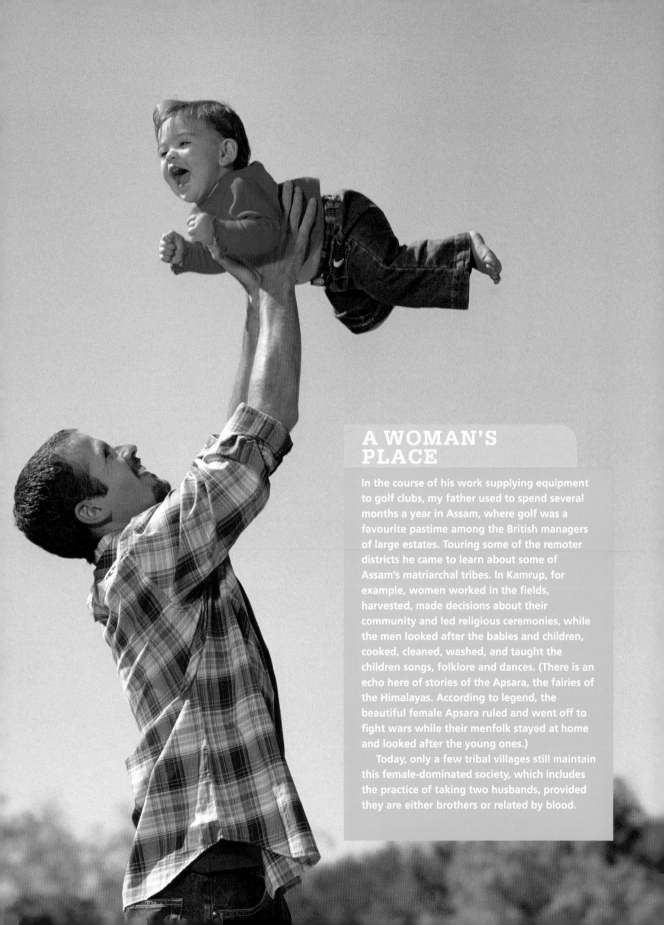

## A WOMAN'S PLACE

In the course of his work supplying equipment to golf clubs, my father used to spend several months a year in Assam, where golf was a favourite pastime among the British managers of large estates. Touring some of the remoter districts he came to learn about some of Assam's matriarchal tribes. In Kamrup, for example, women worked in the fields, harvested, made decisions about their community and led religious ceremonies, while the men looked after the babies and children, cooked, cleaned, washed, and taught the children songs, folklore and dances. (There is an echo here of stories of the Apsara, the fairies of the Himalayas. According to legend, the beautiful female Apsara ruled and went off to fight wars while their menfolk stayed at home and looked after the young ones.)

Today, only a few tribal villages still maintain this female-dominated society, which includes the practice of taking two husbands, provided they are either brothers or related by blood.

Given this background, it seems that the societal distinctions between men and women in terms of rights and power have been man-made. When intellect and mental capacity are compared, it is difficult to find any distinction between the two sexes. If anything, it is boys and men who seem to have the greater struggle and, even within the restrictions of purdah, Middle Eastern universities turn out more women graduates, with higher degrees than men.

So, if not intellectually, where do these differences lie, beyond the obvious physical ones, and how may these affect a woman's health and well-being? Recognizing the deep and very real differences is a step towards improvements for everyone, especially women.

## Skeleto-muscular system

Watch any of the popular archaeological programmes on television nowadays, and you will see skeletons being identified by gender and age. The body is built for the functions it carries out. Most people know that women's hips are wider than men's to make childbirth easier, but a woman's body has a further refinement on this. Just before the baby is due, hormones in the placenta trigger a calcium loss that causes the relevant joints to 'de-fuse', helping the baby pass through without any hitch.

Female bones are also more prone generally to loss of calcium, however, leading to a greater prevalence of osteoporosis (brittle-bone disease), polymyalgia rheumatica (general body aches), cramps in the toes and legs, rheumatoid arthritis and osteoarthritis. It also means that a woman's bones fracture more easily and, if there are serious hormonal problems or a chronic disease such as diabetes, she will generally heal more slowly.

The muscular system develops according to the genetic structure of the body, developed over millions of years. Men therefore tend towards a V shape, with broad shoulders narrowing to the hips, whereas women are the opposite, with less emphasis on the shoulders and wider at the hips.

Women gymnasts, ice skaters and ballerinas are more flexible and graceful than their male counterparts because their structure allows them that freedom, but men have the edge in a performance that demands muscular strength. Unless specially trained, women do not have powerful biceps, calves, pectorals, or abdominal or shoulder muscles. Body-building and extensive sports training alter this, but at a price. The muscle bulk-building hormones in the body are by nature similar to androgens or male hormones, and in excess cause the female body to change – lack of periods and infertility are common problems for exercise instructors, athletes and other women who undergo intensive muscle-building and training. (Anabolic steroids were an extreme example of this, a notorious part of the international sports scene for many years, endowing female athletes with male characteristics such as facial hair as well as the ability to build muscle bulk.)

## SOME DISEASES AND CONDITIONS PREVALENT IN WOMEN

*(There is information on most of these in Part 3.)*

- **migraine** women are affected three times as often as men, and attacks often arise just before or during periods
- **anaemia** about three times more common in women; pregnant women and teenage girls especially prone
- **candidiasis** men can transmit, but most problematic for women
- **urinary tract infection (cystitis)** women's shorter urethra means that infection can reach the bladder more easily
- **rheumatoid arthritis** approximately three times more common in women
- **Sjögren's syndrome** an auto-immune disease that attacks women about nine times as often as men
- **cellulite** deposits of white fat in areas such as the thighs; this is related to conversion and storage of excess hormones, and is much more common in women

- **water retention** swollen ankles and puffy hands occur more frequently in women, and is a condition that occurs especially before periods, in extreme heat and on long flights
- **irritable bowel syndrome (IBS)** afflicts over twice as many women as men
- **polymyalgia rheumatica (PMR)** (general aches in the body) about twice as many women suffer than men
- **scoliosis (curvature of the spine)** occurs about twice as frequently in women
- **lupus** 90 per cent of cases are found in women

On the other hand, men suffer more frequently from kidney stones and tumours, gout, and gastric and duodenal ulcers. More men than women suffer from chronic leukaemia, and about three times as many get the more common form of ankylosing spondylitis, a progressive auto-immune disease in which the hip joints and also the vertebrae in the spine fuse together.

## Blood

The key to all sorts of physical activity is oxygen, carried by blood to the muscles. Proportionate to their size and weight, women have fewer blood cells than men, and a lower volume of blood. It is also slightly thinner. (Menstruation is not a factor in this: menstrual blood is built up over the month in the lining of the womb and its loss has little consequence for the body's general stamina or energy.) A higher proportion of blood, supplying a greater muscle bulk, is what gives men a natural advantage when it comes to power and speed.

Oxygen allows the conversion of glucose to carbon dioxide and water, and so a smaller supply of oxygen will lead more quickly to muscle cramps and fatigue. So, unless specifically developed, women's muscles tire more quickly.

## Digestive system and eating habits

A man's digestive system (in full health) is inclined to be more robust than a woman's as it has evolved to support harder physical work (so it produces more bile, for instance, to cope with greater amounts of food).

Women are more prone to reflect psychological problems in their eating patterns. Eating disorders such as anorexia and bulimia are so much more common among women that they are sometimes wrongly believed to be exclusively a female problem. Stress and bodily changes are also more likely to trigger an alteration in dietary habits: a craving for sweets is common premenstrually, for example, and the cravings of pregnant women can include oddities such as clay or chalk.

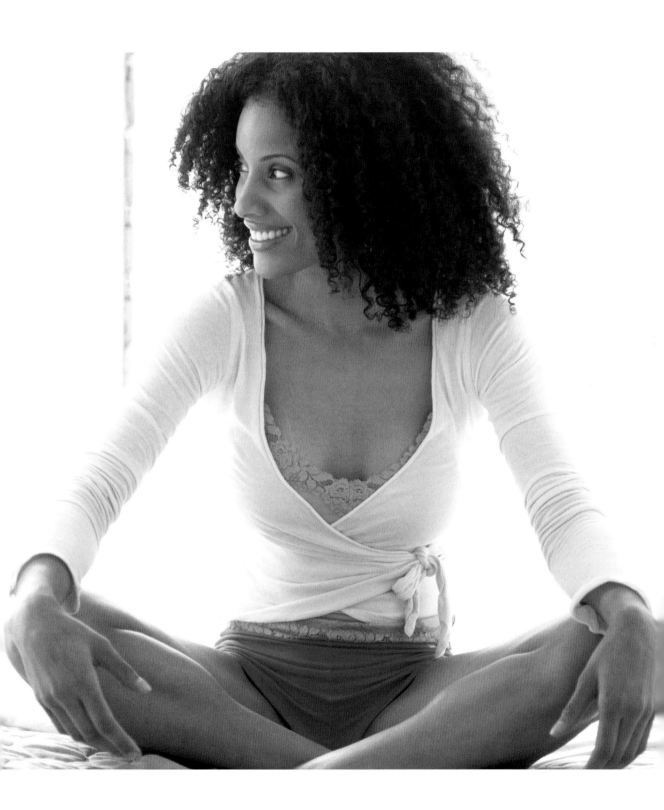

## Mars and Venus

The differences between men and women in their expression of emotions and personality are so great that I sometimes wonder how they can manage to live together – to say that men and women are from different planets is an apt shorthand to express how different they can be in their thinking.

Boys and girls develop and learn differently. Pedagogues are beginning to recognize that part of the problem with boys lagging behind girls academically is that the different 'hard-wiring' of the brain, which is influenced by hormones, means that boys and girls respond differently to certain types of teaching.

Even as young as three years, each sex will tend to seek out its own group to play with and, however strong the conditioning to the contrary, scientific studies have shown a predilection in young boys for playthings that move and work, and a curiosity in exploring, and in girls for toys or activities that involve them in detail or in other people. (This probably relates to boys' faster-developing spatial awareness and girls' more advanced fine motor and observation skills.) These early experiences inevitably contribute to skills and attitudes in later life.

If you grow up with siblings of the opposite sex, you get to learn a bit about each other's habits and behaviour, but if you do not, or if you spend years in a single-sex school, you are often ignorant of the psychological trends of the other sex. In courtship, and as a family, when you look beyond the physical relationship this can lead to great difficulties.

One observation often made by patients I see is that 'He's a different person' or 'She's changed completely'. Shakespeare and others have written about 'the seven

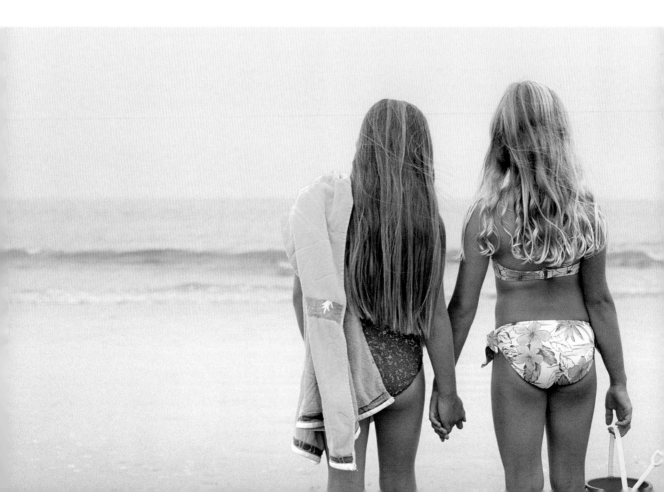

## WHAT MAKES YOU A WOMAN?

We all begin our life as female. The sex chromosomes in our genes – XX for female, XY for male – are there from the moment of conception, but it is only after six weeks of development in the womb that the first secretions of male hormones trigger the initial stages of development into a boy; until then male and female embryos are identical.

In the earliest stages the rudimentary external genitalia look exactly the same in both sexes. Under the influence of male hormones, what is the clitoris in a female becomes the penis in a male, the larger folds of the vagina become the male scrotum and the smaller folds of the vagina become the shaft of the penis. The testes begin to develop in the male abdominal cavity and descend slowly into the scrotum around the time of birth, while in the female the ovaries remain inside, held in place by ligaments so that they do not drop with gravity.

Sometimes, despite the genetic programming, an embryo is not exposed to male hormones at the appropriate time and the reproductive organs will not modify in this way (and the reverse is also true: a genetically female embryo exposed to an excess of male hormones at this time can develop genitalia with male characteristics). Although these intersex conditions are not common they occur more often than is generally realized and indicate that nature, in its infinite variety, is not easily pigeonholed into X or Y.

ages of man', reflecting our progression through growth and maturity to old age. These stages, each with their own characteristics, happen roughly every seven years. Of course, we don't switch overnight from child to adolescent at 14 and adolescent to adult at 21, or hit a mid-life crisis at 56, but there is a discernible rhythm to our lives.

At the beginning and end of life both sexes are similar, but in our middle years in particular the differences in attitude and outlook are particularly noticeable. For a man and woman to continue to live together harmoniously as a couple means constant adjustment and compromise on both sides and an acknowledgement that change is part of life.

## Hormones

A major influence on mood, and therefore outlook on life, is hormones. Both men and women have hormones, of course – after all, they are the deciding factor in whether we are male or female even before we are born – but the hormonal changes in women are more prominent and so the cycles of moods are more noticeable. Premenstrual tension, post-natal depression and behavioural changes in the early stages of pregnancy are some examples of the hormone-induced mood changes in women. Many of the problems and conditions explored in Part 3, from menopausal anxiety to weight control, have a hormonal element.

# Types of women
Since certain characteristics are often seen to fall together, this has led scientists and philosophers down the centuries to devise formulas for grouping people.

Traditional Chinese medicine observes yin and yang aspects of every part of nature, including ourselves, while astrologists have long used the configuration of the stars at our birth as a guide to our personality and fate. In the early twentieth century Jung was separating Introverts from Extroverts, and Pavlov devised the labels Lively, Impetuous, Calm and Weak; and using blood groups to divine people's physical and temperamental type is a more recent trend first popularized in Japan.

In about 500 BC Charaka, the father of ayurvedic medicine, devised three categories into which people could be classified. In recent years ayurveda has gained great popularity in the West and many patients, mostly women, ask me to confirm whether they are vata, pitta or kapha. Although I use and recommend ayurvedic remedies and have learnt much from this ancient approach to health and healing, it can be deceptive to adhere too unquestioningly to these traditional categories. The guidance given for balancing overwhelmingly pitta traits, for instance, was to consume extra sugar, but nowadays our bodies are more prone than in the past to an excess of yeasts and fungal overgrowth, so adding more sugar will compound the problem, whichever category you may fall into.

## WHAT'S YOUR STAR SIGN?

Scientifically speaking, there is no proof that the planets influence the course of our lives, yet millions around the world read their horoscopes daily and, for many, asking someone their star sign is a way of finding out about their personality.

Arguing about how planets may affect our lives is not the intention of this book. But if tides are affected by the moon, and plant and animal life by the sun, might the planets and stars not have an effect on us? Whether it is based on knowledge read in the heavens or simply intuition fortified by experience, a good astrologer's details of character analysis are often amazingly accurate.

In India, it is customary to make a birth chart soon after a child is born. This is kept by pandits, learned priests trained in astrology, whose guidance is sought in making the right choices in life. Even educated and cosmopolitan Indians will consult the stars before launching a new business, releasing a film in Bollywood, recruiting staff or choosing a date for a journey.

Analysing birth charts is an essential part of Indian matchmaking. Astrologers pay special attention to manglikas, those born under the influence of Mars, because they have a strange fate: they can never remain married for long except to another manglika. I have also noted inexplicable influences of gemstones associated with specific star signs. One patient had had headaches and panic attacks from the time her husband had given her a diamond ring. When, after a minor squabble, she did not wear it for some time, amazingly all her ailments disappeared. She told me about it and I asked her to wear it again. She was soon back at the clinic for treatment. She never wore that ring again. Perhaps coincidence, but I have had other patients, both men and women, whom certain stones did not suit.

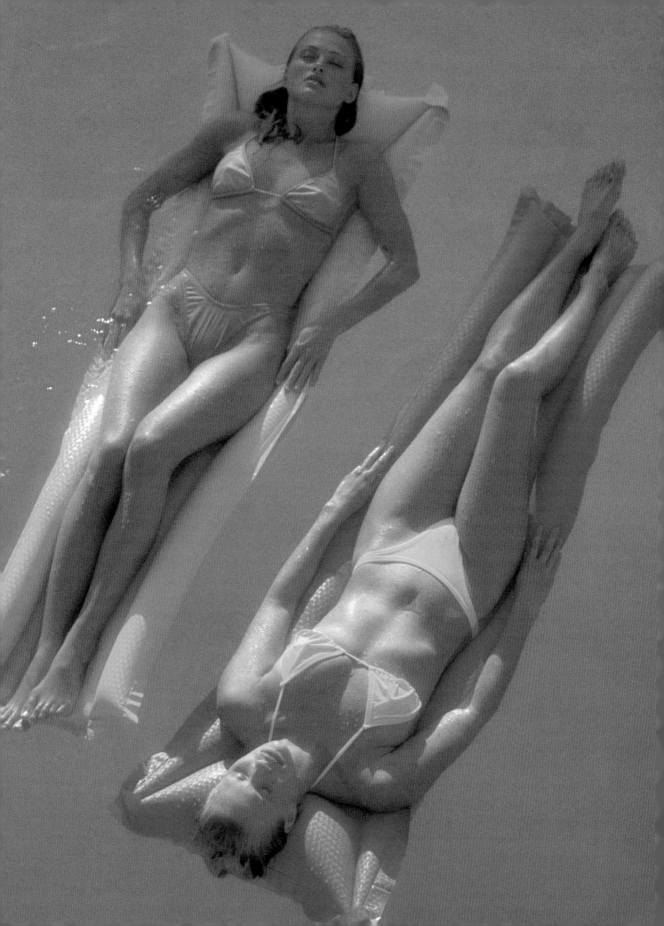

# The four humours

It is also often forgotten that for centuries the West had its own form of classification by type. Galen, the renowned Greek physician who lived in the second century AD, categorized people according to the balance and influence within them of the four humours: blood (sanguine), bile (choleric), phlegm (phlegmatic) and black bile (melancholic).

His system continued to be widely used for diagnosis and treatment for over 1,500 years, and I have found that, even despite the changes in society, ways of living and medical advances, his experience and detailed observation often holds good today. You may find the following interesting. Most women will find they are a mixture, usually of two types. If you are 50 per cent or more true to one type then you could classify yourself in that category.

## SANGUINE WOMEN

- Well-built, tall and muscular; good volume of dark, straight hair.
- Athletic, love sport and the challenge of competition. The physical and mental stamina to compete with men, and as girls might have been called tomboys.
- Bad losers, often brooding or crying over losing, but bouncing back next time, perhaps to perform even better.
- Can experience intense anger but calm down quickly; will often apologize very tactfully without fully accepting they were wrong.
- Speak fast, blink more frequently than average and quick in answering questions, often before the question is complete. Witty and often challenging in conversation or debates. Like being listened to and often find others' ideas or speech boring. Theirs is often the last word.
- Optimistic and always see light at the end of the tunnel.
- Courageous, often taking calculated risks to solve problems, but great softness when hurt. Failure or bereavement hit particularly badly, and they take longer to get over hurt or betrayal. Once out of it, they regain their strength.
- Leadership qualities, attracting men and women to follow their ideas.

**Family and relationships:**
- Attract weaker men ready to do anything they are asked.
- Motherhood brings out softer side.
- Often excellent with children, good at handling discipline and instilling principles.

**Reproductive health:**
- Good, regular menstrual periods.
- Conceive easily unless they exercise excessively.

**General health:**
- High level of activity means weight gain seldom a worry.
- Eat fast and digest well.
- Can consume more alcohol than other women without after-effects.
- May suffer headaches and have a tendency to high blood pressure.
- Suffer few colds or coughs and heal well.
- Sleep easily and get up fresh. Often dream of disaster.

## CHOLERIC WOMEN

- Tall and well built, stockier than sanguine women.
- Light, soft skin with clear eyes, often blue or green, and curly hair that is often dark.
- Graceful, soft spoken and careful about what they say.
- Tend to hide feelings and if they do cry, they do so in private.
- Fairly active and exercise regularly from concern about their figure even though weight tends not to be problematic.
- Vigilant and often cunning; good at arguing their point but decision-making may be slow (compared to sanguine).
- Good memory.

### Family and relationships:

- Sensitive; can get hurt very badly.
- Can find themselves in unstable relationships.

### Reproductive health:

- Good menstrual flow and regular periods, but may be painful or be accompanied by migraines (usually one or the other, rarely both).
- Suffer from premenstrual mood fluctuations, bloating and water retention; they become irritable and argumentative as they are intelligent women who hate to suddenly lose their logic and coolness once a month.
- Conceive easily but have digestive problems in early and late pregnancy (bad morning sickness) and can gain a fair amount of weight.
- Good volume of breast milk and happy to nurse babies for a long time.

### General health:

There is a saying: 'God gives beauty to some women but also gives many illnesses and problems.' This is most applicable to choleric women.

- Inclined to sweat a lot and may have strong body odour, making them very conscious of personal hygiene.
- Good appetite but trouble digesting oily, rich, spicy or heavy food, making them cautious eaters as digestion problems may follow.
- Very conscious of abdominal bloating, heartburn, alternating constipation with diarrhoea, all symptoms of irritable bowels.
- Careful eating keeps weight under check, but abdominal bloating may give impression of a thick waist.
- Digestive problems may result in bad breath.
- Generally bad sleepers, suffering from fatigue and lethargy.
- More likely to suffer from skin problems such as eczema, acne, dandruff or dry skin.
- Aching joints may restrict activity.

## PHLEGMATIC WOMEN

- Often referred to as 'fat, fair and flabby'. Straight, usually thin, light-coloured hair and fair skin that is cold and moist to touch, with bluish veins often visible.
- Muscles hidden away under a layer of fat and usually less developed.
- Very conscious of weight and often camouflage it with good clothes and jewellery, of which they are very fond.
- Draw people to them with their great personal charm.

◆ Come across as cheerful, funny and happy-go-lucky, but hide their feelings well and can be very insecure and sensitive – they can make the whole world laugh while crying inside. Their weight may make them secretly depressed.

◆ Often uncertain of themselves; influenced by what people say and may consult clairvoyants and others for opinions and guidance.

### Family and relationships:

◆ Set great store by their families.

◆ Caring by nature and always help those who need it most. Very charitable and concerned about the poor and suffering.

◆ Love to cook and feed others (and may snack frequently even though they claim not to eat much).

### Reproductive health:

◆ Periods typically light and often irregular.

◆ More likely than other types to suffer from polycystic ovaries, endometriosis, infertility, excess body hair or low thyroid function, indicating hormonal problems.

### General health:

◆ Intolerant of heat and cold; can have cold hands and feet even in summer.

◆ Low blood pressure and sluggish metabolism.

◆ Constipation can be a problem, so haemorrhoids, varicose veins, water retention and swollen ankles are common complaints.

◆ General aches and pains in joints and more prone to fractures and sprains.

◆ Bruise easily and often have brittle nails due to calcium deficiency (perhaps due to constipation). They also get cramp in their toes and calves at night.

◆ Tend to suffer from gallstones, diabetes and sinus or bronchial problems.

◆ Can also suffer from depression and eating disorders such as bulimia.

◆ Usually very concerned about their health and will consult various therapists and doctors.

◆ Sleep well but often get up tired. Dreams seem lengthy and vivid and frequently involve water.

## MELANCHOLIC WOMEN

◆ Typically, thin, not very tall, and with poorly developed muscles; may have poor posture.

◆ Often creative in the fields of writing or art.

◆ May be very religious and like reading spiritual books.

◆ Soft spoken and calm, listening more than they talk; it takes a lot to make them angry.

◆ Tend to keep their problems to themselves and rarely speak their mind.

◆ The pessimists of this world, always seeing the darker side of life, as if they are wearing dark glasses all the time. Depression, insomnia and anxiety are often problems as a consequence.

### Family and relationships:

◆ Caring nature makes them good mothers; they will be inclined to read books and to take much advice on childcare.

◆ Derive great strength and pleasure from their children and, as they are not interfering parents (perhaps rather too soft and kind), give children the sort of freedom they love.

◆ May be keen for their children to grow up differently from themselves.

## Reproductive health:

◆ Inclined to light or scanty periods lasting just two or three days on average.

◆ May have fertility problems, or find pregnancy a struggle or fraught with complications, perhaps linked to nutritional problems.

## General health:

◆ Often shun too much meat and feel better with vegetables or fish; many are vegetarians.

◆ Constipation, bloating and heartburn can be problems. Poor appetite and digestion makes them inclined to eat the same type of food most of the time and be afraid to experiment with new foods.

◆ Inclined to low blood pressure, dry skin and very cold hands and feet from poor circulation (chilblains are a frequent complaint).

◆ Other tendencies include rheumatoid arthritis, osteoarthritis, hair loss, osteoporosis and chronic fatigue syndrome.

◆ Worry about health can lead towards hypochondria.

Although, like fingerprints, every individual is different, people do share common traits. Genes dictate our basic underlying type, but geographical origin, diet, religion, culture and lifestyle all affect our appearance, behaviour and way of thinking. They influence what we eat and our attitude to body shape, our state of health and predisposition to certain illnesses, even our expectations from life.

# A VIEW FROM THE EAST

After much trouble, a bookseller in Rajasthan found for me, from a private library, a tattered copy of an ancient book on man–woman relationships. In it I discovered that even a couple of thousand years ago there was a fascination with classifying people by type, and links were being drawn between physical build, psyche, behavioural pattern and predisposition towards particular illnesses. The book describes four types of women in typically picturesque language …

Padmini (lotus type) … She has the lustre and splendour of a lotus flower … her skin is as fair as the jasmine … she is quite reserved, very loyal to her friends, family and husband … she may suffer frequently from headaches, menstrual problems and digestive disorders but is able to regain her strength quickly.

Chitrini (picture like) … Her breasts and hips are large but her feet are small … she loves to sing and is extremely fond of music, dance and art … she is easily aroused sexually and likes to be touched and caressed … she is generally healthy but may suffer from weight problems and joint problems.

Shankhini (conch like) … Her eyes are big and she has a long face … she knows about the ways of the world … she is often very short-tempered … she has digestive problems and suffers from headaches, arthritis and liver disease.

Hastini (elephant like) … She is fat and often short, with large hips and thighs … her toes are often thick and crooked … she is a great matriarch, controlling everybody in the family … she has joint and back pain, breathing difficulties and often sluggish bowels.

# optimum health

The basic aim of my Lifestyle Programme is to arouse the physis or healing power within the body and nurture it. It has been inspired by Hippocrates' regimen therapy (described in Part 1) and formulated to cover all aspects of maintenance of health and well-being.

I have used the Lifestyle Programme as a tool to combat and prevent illness and to restore health in thousands of patients in the past 20 years or so. It might be described as a cure-all, since whether the problem is hormonal, stress-related, digestive, circulatory, muscular or other,

# part 2

the method to treat and cure it remains the same. For those who hate taking medicines or believe in self-help, this is an ideal programme, as it works by helping the body's innate forces to regulate and enhance healing.

But first, I advise you to embark on some self-testing with an MOT (My Own Testing). This will help you to assess your state of health and well-being, think about any problems or weaknesses you may have and how they might relate to your lifestyle. It may also help you view your state of health as being more than just 'not ill'.

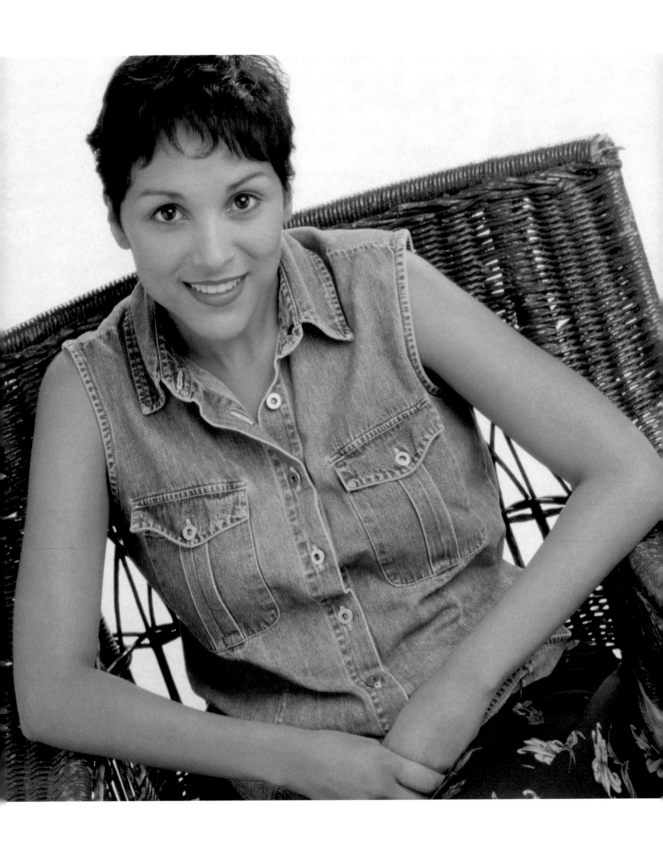

# chapter one

# giving yourself an MOT

MOT, or My Own Testing, is designed to help you get to know your own body better. By observing how it works when you're feeling good and not so good, how it reacts to different situations, pressures and foods, and attuning yourself to its rhythms, you will be able to pick up the early-warning signs that anything might be amiss and take steps to regain optimum health before things go seriously wrong.

# The overall picture Work through the following checklist to assess your general state of health. Then try following the Lifestyle Programme and return to the MOT every six weeks or couple of months to see what improvements you have noticed.

If you recognize any of the following in yourself, or if your answers to any of the questions highlight a specific concern, follow the relevant recommendations in Part 3. If your condition does not improve within a month, then you must consult an appropriately qualified physician.

## Weight

In the chapter on Weight Control is a chart that explains how to work out your body mass index (BMI), as a guide to your optimum weight. The BMI is still only a guideline, and doesn't take into account bones lightened by osteoporosis or distinguish fat from muscle (muscle is heavier). It is, however, a useful starting point.

At the same time as you weigh yourself, measure your waist. Keep a note of it so that you can see whether your waist is steadily increasing (allowing for anything such as temporary abdominal bloating).

Weight is not just a matter of measurements, it's how it affects your sense of well-being and level of activity. You probably weigh too much if:

◆ you have had to move up a dress size, or your skirts and trousers have become tight round the waist
◆ you get breathless walking up a flight of stairs
◆ you get backache when exercising, standing around or even just sitting

◆ you often feel lethargic or sluggish, especially in the morning
◆ your groin, just above the pubic bone, feels very sore (press it and check).

If your BMI suggests you are underweight, check whether you have some or all of the following confirming indications:

◆ your hands and feet feel cold very easily
◆ you get frequent colds and coughs (immune system is weak)
◆ you lose hair very easily
◆ you bruise easily and/or your nails flake
◆ your appetite and/or your digestion are poor
◆ your joints and body ache.

Weighing yourself too often isn't helpful – it can either be discouraging if you are trying to lose weight but it isn't coming off as quickly as you would like, or you can get obsessional about small gains or losses of 1kg or less. Every couple of months is enough unless you are worried by a sudden rise or drop in your size.

Dramatic weight loss is not healthy, nor is a fluctuating weight, which is often the result of yo-yo dieting. If your body doesn't know where the next meal is coming from it will go into 'famine' mode, storing even more fat and conserving energy, causing you to slow down in both body and mind.

## Eating and drinking habits

- How many portions of fruit and vegetables do you eat every day?
- Do you eat meat: at almost every meal, every day, once or twice a week, less often or never?
- How many times a week do you eat fish?
- The diet section of the Lifestyle Programme has information on nutrients that are particularly vital for women. Does your diet include all of these in sufficient quantities?
- Do you always have breakfast?
- Is your main meal of the day at lunchtime or in the evening?
- Are you a habitual snacker?
- Do you quite often (at least once a week, on average) get up in the middle of the night for a snack?
- Do you drink about 1½–2 litres of water a day?
- Do you drink more than the recommended amount of alcohol a week (see box below)?

What, when and how you eat and drink affects not only your weight (see chapter on Weight Control) but your general performance, including the alertness of your mind. The various chapters in Part 3 also explain how adjusting your diet can help counteract particular problems.

## Digestion

- Do you have a bowel movement every day? Your bowels should move at least once every 24 hours or so. Chronic constipation can be an indication of several health problems, and can also create them.
- Do you experience excessive burping or wind? Do you feel bloated after meals? This can be an indication of an over-acidic stomach (see pages 56–7) or other digestive disturbance, or stress.
- Your urine should be a clear, pale yellow. If it is a stronger yellow, or dark, you are probably not drinking enough fluids.

## ALCOHOL INTAKE

Recommendations for maximum alcohol intake for a woman vary between 14 and 21 units a week. People often kid themselves that 1 drink = 1 unit, but this is not so:

- 1 bar measure of average wine = 1½ units (home measures are often 2 units)
- 1 bar measure (25 ml) of spirits or fortified wines = 1 unit (home measures are often 2 or 3 units)
- ½ pint cider or lager = 1 unit

The high number of units in cocktails is often overlooked if their alcoholic content is masked by cream or fruit.

It is not advisable to drink alcohol while you are pregnant or trying to get pregnant.

Remember that alcohol is also high in calories, so if you are trying to lose weight (see part 3, chapter seven, Weight Control) then you should also watch what you drink. Light spirits like gin and vodka, and champagne and white wine are lower in calories than beer, red wine and fortified wines, which in addition to their calorific content are also more likely to cause digestive problems.

◆ Does your urine smell strongly? This may indicate an excess of vitamins (particularly B) or protein.

◆ Do you have a burning sensation as you pass urine? This may be a sign of cystitis, or you may not be drinking enough water, or your diet may be too highly spiced or acidic.

◆ Cup your hands over your mouth and nose. Breathe out deeply through your mouth and then breathe in through your nose. A smell like nail varnish is caused by excess yeast and fermenting alcohol in the stomach (see pages 58–9). An ammoniacal smell (like bad eggs) indicates putrefaction. It could be caused by excess protein, failure to digest properly, or from problem gums.

# Heart and lungs

## BLOOD PRESSURE

High blood pressure can be related to a number of health problems, including 'furred' arteries and living in a state of heightened stress, and it can increase the risk of heart attack, stroke, thrombosis and other health threats.

The heart is, basically, a pump, and blood pressure is given as two figures: systolic (higher) and diastolic (lower), which are the different readings as the heart contracts and relaxes. When you are at rest your blood pressure levels should be between 120/70 and 135/85, although blood pressure tends to rise with age, and up to 150/90 can be considered normal if you are over 60. A diastolic pressure of below 60 or above 90 is outside the normal range at any age.

Have your blood pressure checked regularly. You can do this at home yourself (although it is not always easy to get an accurate reading from meters sold to the public) or go to a drop-in clinic or a pharmacy that offers the facility. Many surgeries will check your blood pressure as a matter of course whatever you might be visiting for, in order to be alerted by tell-tale changes.

## PULSE

How fast your heart beats is another indication of how hard it is having to work. When at rest around 60–75 beats per minute is normal. If you are very fit it may be slower than this, as the heart, along with other muscles, becomes more efficient with regular exercise.

Try checking your pulse before you start an exercise period and then immediately afterwards (when it will have speeded up from the demands you have placed on your body) and then every five minutes or so as your body relaxes, to see how quickly your pulse returns to normal.

To measure your pulse, use a watch that counts seconds. Place three fingers of one hand across the inner wrist of the other hand, just below the base of the thumb. Ensure you can feel your pulse clearly. If it is over 80 when you are relaxed and rested, or you discern any irregularity, go and get it checked by a health professional.

## BREATHING

Put your hand on top of your abdomen and check you're breathing normally (it's easy to pant or hold your breath when you make yourself conscious of your breathing). Time your in-breaths for a minute. If the rate is much above 16 per minute you are hyperventilating – this could be a nervous reaction (test yourself several times), or it could mean that excess abdominal gas is lifting the diaphragm and not leaving you enough room to breathe deeply. It may also indicate a heart or lung problem.

# Energy levels

As well as using up our energy supply in the obvious way, with physical activity, we also use up a surprising amount simply running our internal systems – thinking and digesting both consume a lot of energy – and with worry or tension.

**Energy check:**

◆ When you wake in the morning do you feel refreshed and ready to greet the day?

◆ Do you still feel sluggish even after you have showered and dressed?

◆ By mid-afternoon do you still feel energetic, or do you feel that typical after-lunch lethargy hitting you?

◆ Does a reasonable, but not highly strenuous, amount of exercise (say half an hour's brisk walk or swim, or a dance class) leave you feeling invigorated or exhausted?

◆ How many hours a night do you usually sleep?

◆ Do you suffer from broken or interrupted sleep more than a couple of times a week?

◆ Has your sleep pattern changed recently?

Lack of energy is like a power 'burn-out' – if our energy is low, then everything burns more dimly. Feeling tired after a full day is natural, but regular exhaustion, especially if you are not doing much, suggests one or more of the following:

◆ you are not getting enough fuel (too little food, or too little of the right sort of food, or trouble with absorbing the goodness from what you are eating)

◆ your energy is being sapped by nervous tension

◆ your body is having to draw on more energy than usual to process food or repair itself (which is why most forms of illness leave you feeling listless and with no 'get up and go')

◆ poor sleep or lack of sleep is not giving your body a chance to recharge its energy reserves.

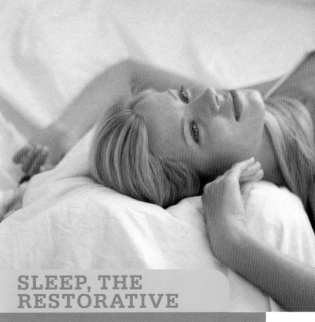

## SLEEP, THE RESTORATIVE

There is no hard-and-fast rule about how much sleep we need, and each individual is different; many elderly people find they need less sleep than they did when they were younger, perhaps because they are expending less energy. But less than four hours' sleep a night on a regular basis is not conducive to good health, and most people function best if they get six or seven hours of refreshing sleep at least three or four nights a week.

If you are ill, then long hours of sleep are a great part of the healing process, and teenagers benefit from more sleep than average (growing and the demands of studying and exams take their toll, as well as the inevitable late nights). But otherwise, feeling you need, say, ten hours or more of sleep a night may indicate a problem such as depression or chronic fatigue.

Sleep doesn't necessarily have to be taken all at one go. A half-hour siesta after lunch is very energizing (see page 250), and if you are breastfeeding or looking after very young children you should take every chance you can to give yourself some restorative sleep.

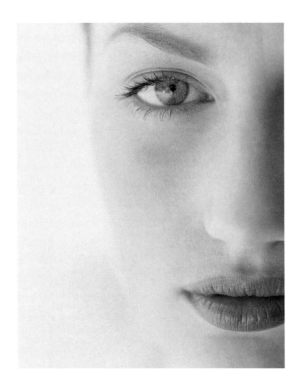

Do you also suffer from heartburn or indigestion? High stomach acid can also result in dry skin.

If none of these seems to provide the answer, it could be a vitamin deficiency. Try the ancient practice of putting mustard oil under your toenails, and massage it into your palms and the soles of your feet. Goodness knows how your body distributes it, but it really does help to alleviate dryness in those areas.

### Do you suffer from an over-oily or greasy skin?

This occurs when the sebaceous glands in the skin are working overtime to eliminate fat-soluble toxins. This can be because of an excess that needs to be disposed of, or because, for example, constipation is preventing elimination by other means. Over-excited sebaceous glands can also upset the uppermost layer of skin, causing it to become itchy or scaly or over-oily.

### Check also for any of the following signs:

- red nose (not from cold weather, an allergy, or a cold): an indicator of too much yeast in your system, or too much alcohol
- itchy skin: can be due to excessive garlic or salt, or to citric or acidic foods, such as vinegar or pineapple
- darker pigment patches on face (particularly noticeable after exposure to the sun): this is chloasma (see page 164)
- soreness at the corners of the mouth: a possible vitamin deficiency, particularly of vitamins A and B
- quantities of bluish white spots on arms, legs and body: indicates high stomach acid and hyperactivity of the pancreas. Eating too much too fast can lead to these marks
- brownish patches on the cheeks: chronic anaemia or liver malfunction.

## Skin, hair and nails

### SKIN

**Is your skin usually dry?**
This may be caused by washing away natural oils or by a dietary deficiency.

- Are you bathing in over-hot water, thereby removing too much of the skin's natural lubrication?
- Might the soap or skin cleanser you're using be too harsh, or do you scrub too fiercely with a loofah?
- How much oil are you consuming in your diet? If sufficient, perhaps your liver is not digesting it properly. Oil needs to be balanced, not too much or too little – a maximum of 4 tablespoons of olive oil in cooking per day is a useful rule of thumb.

## HAIR

Your hair, like your skin, is a reflection of inner health. If you are ill, or chronically below par or stressed, this shows in dull, out-of-condition hair. Check also for the following:

◆ a sudden increase in hair loss: this could indicate a nutritional deficiency, a hormonal imbalance, stress or trauma, low blood pressure, or other restriction that means the scalp is not getting as much oxygenated blood as it should. (Thinning hair is also common in older women; see pages 289–90.)

◆ hair falling out in patches: this could be alopecia, a fungal infection or auto-immune problem

◆ dandruff or flaking scalp: sebaceous glands working overtime (see above)

◆ dry, itchy scalp not caused by dandruff: may be due to zinc deficiency.

Diagnostic hair testing is a good indicator of any past deficiency of minerals but doesn't necessarily reflect your current state of health.

## NAILS

Nails take about four months to grow from the base to the top, so they provide a history of your recent state of health. Study your nails periodically to see what they tell you:

◆ horizontal ridge or indentation: an interruption in the nail's growth, reflecting an interruption in your health. (Where it occurs indicates how long ago it was, so halfway up your nail would be about two months ago.) A series of such bands would indicate a long period or recurrent problem that may still be ongoing

◆ white patches: a mineral deficiency (though not necessarily of calcium, as is commonly believed; zinc is more likely)

◆ vertical streaks: a sign of ongoing chronic disease.

# Eyes

Looking carefully at your eyes can help you gauge the state of your health.

◆ Tenseness will slightly shrivel the small blood vessels in the sclera (the white portion)

◆ A long period of stress (which may include sleeplessness) or an overload of toxins in the system will cause these blood vessels to burst. If this has happened recently the eyes will appear bloodshot

◆ If the situation continues the iron in the blood will turn the white of the eye yellow-brown (just like a scab on your skin). Definitely time you took remedial action.

# Tongue

An experienced physician can diagnose various conditions of the body by inspecting the tongue, including anaemia, dehydration, presence of gut yeast or fungus, constipation, acidity, liver malfunction and stomach ulcers. Here are some signs you can look for:

◆ Is it furry at the back? This indicates excessive acid or that you are not evacuating toxins well enough (perhaps because of constipation).

◆ Does it have a smooth narrow red band round the edge? Another sign of excess acidity.

◆ Any small ulcerations or cracks, particularly in the middle? These may mean your liver is sluggish or you have excess yeast in the gut.

◆ Is the tip reddish? You are eating too many carbohydrates.

◆ Does it look slightly shrivelled and shiny? You are not drinking enough water.

◆ Are there impressions of the teeth either side? Gastric upsets can expand your tongue so much that it presses against the sides of the teeth.

# Health through the years As Part 3 explains in detail, your age is a key factor in identifying particular areas of concern.

In addition to the general monitoring of your health, there are things you should be especially aware of at different stages in your life.

## If you are in your teens or twenties

- When considering methods of contraception, find out about the pros and cons of each (see page 132–7). Don't feel obliged to stick with the first method you are recommended, or the one your friend finds best.
- Chlamydia is an increasing worry among young women, as it so often goes undetected (see page 139).
- It is never too young to start protecting your skin against damage and premature ageing (not only from the sun but the environment in general) and your bones against osteoporosis.
- Anorexia hits teenage girls more than anyone else. Be alert to any early signs of it in anyone vulnerable and close to you, such as a daughter or younger sister (see pages 258–61).
- Ensure you get enough sleep. Particularly in your early teens you are still growing, and intensive studying is a big drain on your energy. If you are a young mother, sleep deprivation can lead to real health problems.

## If you are in your thirties or forties

- Once a month check your breasts for any changes or lumps (see page 198).
- Have a regular cervical smear and vaginal check-up (usually about every one to three years) to detect any pre-cancerous cell development.
- Demands on your time and energy will probably never be higher, especially if you are a working mother. Guard against becoming run down as this will make you vulnerable to health problems.
- Review any method of contraception you are using, to ensure it is the most suitable for you and your circumstances.
- Increasingly, women are waiting until their thirties or even forties to have children, but fertility starts to decline after about the age of 35.

## If you are in your fifties

- Some women welcome the menopause and others dread it, but there is much you can do to alleviate the symptoms (see part 3, chapter eleven, Ageing Gracefully).
- Weight gain can be a problem in your forties and fifties when it never was before; this may be linked to a change in lifestyle or a slowing metabolism, or may be hormonal in origin.

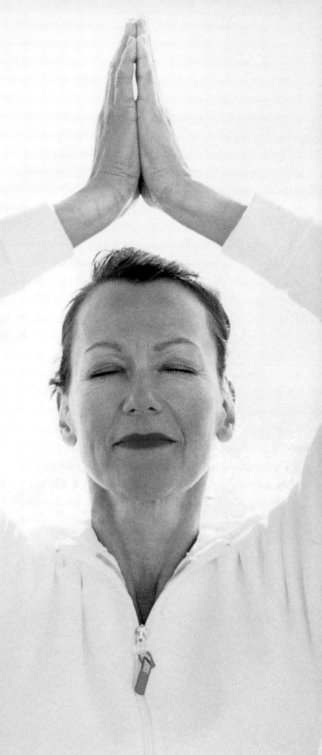

- A sensible exercise regime will help keep weight in check and keep bones strong against osteoporosis.
- Your hair and skin are both likely to be drier and less resilient than a decade ago, so ensure you are using the most appropriate moisturizers and shampoos.
- Continue monthly breast checks and take advantage of mammogram checks (usually every three years).

## If you are in your sixties, or over

- Review your eating habits. Both women and men in their sixties find their digestion becomes more sluggish and less tolerant of certain foods. Having smaller meals (especially in the evening) and avoiding the 'baddies' described on page 305 often help avoid the digestive problems from which so many older people suffer. Chronic constipation, for example, is not only uncomfortable but injurious to bones and joints as it impairs calcium absorption.
- Keep an eye on your weight: you should neither gain a lot nor lose a lot – being too fat puts pressure on your joints and makes you less mobile, while being too skinny can mean you feel the cold more and are also more vulnerable to osteoporosis.
- Regular exercise such as yoga or tai chi will help keep you supple without straining muscles and joints.

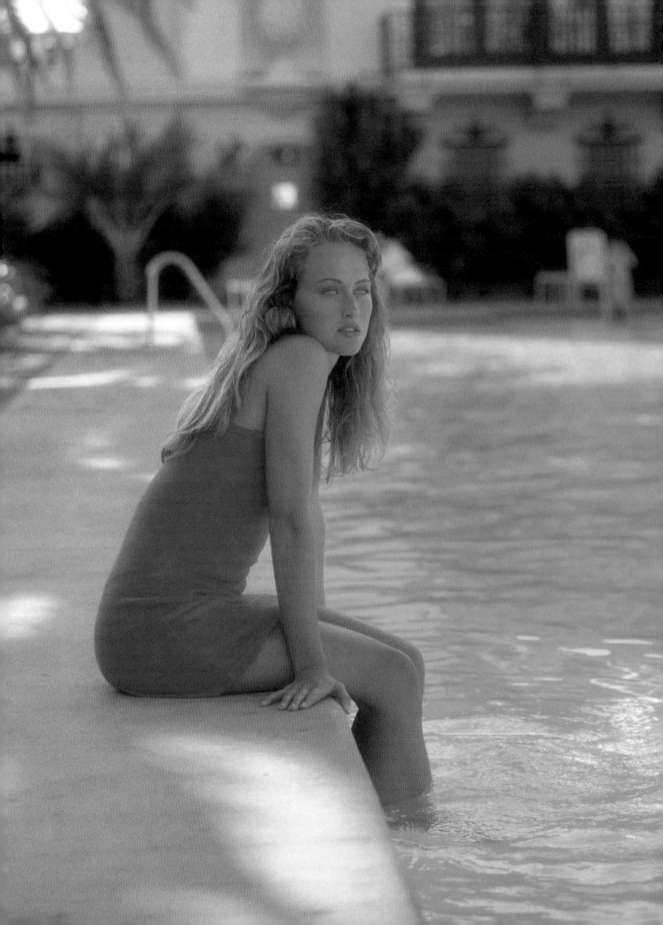

# Life balance You should candidly review the balance between four key areas in your life: exercise, stress, relaxation and moderation.

## Exercise

◆ How regularly do you exercise?
◆ Is it giving you a good workout without straining you? If you suffer from cramps you are probably overdoing it.
◆ Does an exercise session leave you feeling invigorated and feeling good, or totally exhausted?
◆ Does the exercise you get make you sleep better at night?

## Stress

◆ Would you describe your life as highly stressed? (This is not the same as busy, but a life that leaves you frequently or constantly feeling you are under unwelcome pressure, or not coping, or straining to keep up appearances.)
◆ How well do you cope with decision-making?
◆ Do you thrive on conflict or are you upset by it?
◆ How do you cope with unexpected change?
◆ When did you last cry with laughter?

## Relaxation

◆ When did you last have a holiday?
◆ Are your holidays very different from your everyday life, or much the same in a different location?
◆ How often do you have a massage?
◆ How often do you sit down to listen to music (i.e. devote your attention to it, not just having the radio on while you're ironing, getting supper or writing a report), or to do something quietly creative, such as painting, modelling or reading for pleasure?
◆ Do you switch off when you get home from work, or do you bring work – or worry about work – home with you?

## Moderation

◆ Are there certain areas of your life that dominate?
◆ Do people call you a workaholic?
◆ Do you have a life independent of your partner or children?
◆ When did you last learn or do something quite new and different?

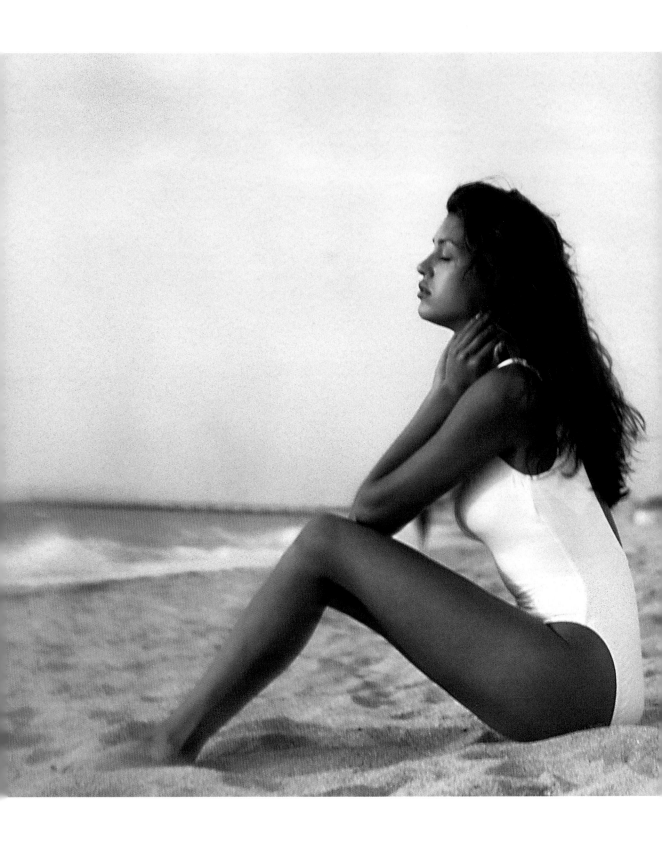

# chapter two

# the lifestyle programme

The three essentials of my general Lifestyle Programme have always been diet, massage and yoga or other exercise. Women often face more emotional and psychological stresses, so I have introduced a greater emphasis on the relaxation element of the programme, and I have also taken into account the fact that problems among my patients often stem from doing things to excess, be it eating or exercising or taking on responsibilities. This Lifestyle Programme, tailored to women, therefore consists of nutrition, massage, exercise (yoga in particular), relaxation and moderation.

The Lifestyle Programme may be quite difficult to follow throughout life, as it requires some discipline. Some people find the dietary guidelines no restriction at all, while others do find them a struggle, especially if their diet until now has relied heavily on convenience food or eating out or satisfying strong cravings.

My suggestion is that if you have any health problems, you should follow the guidelines strictly for four to six months (hormonal problems will take about this time to become regulated). After that, you can keep to the general guidelines but allow yourself more latitude. Once or twice a year, go back to the programme for a few weeks whenever you judge your general well-being may have dipped. Many people find it useful to put this programme into practice between January and March, after the excesses of Christmas, and then again after their summer holiday or a time at work that has been particularly hard.

The longer you can follow the regime, the easier it will become and the less you will want to revert to bad old ways. Once you have discovered how your body reacts when it is functioning optimally, you will never want to go back.

# Nutrition
Everyone knows they should eat healthily, but people have different ideas about what this means; and it is not always recognized that everyone – and women in particular – should adjust their diet according to their circumstances.

You may routinely be given nutritional advice while pregnant or breastfeeding, but adapting your diet is important at many other times, including the different stages of the menstrual cycle, at puberty, at the menopause and in old age.

## My approach to nutrition

To remain healthy we all need protein, carbohydrates and fats in appropriate quantities and proportions, plus all the vitamins and minerals our bodies need, and water. Restrictions and commands that forbid you from eating specific foodstuffs lead you to look at food in the wrong way. If you follow the general guidance given in this section, aim for moderation and learn to listen to your body, you are unlikely to go wrong.

Many of women's major areas of concern about health – periods, skin, weight, emotions, energy, fertility, well-being – can be influenced by diet. Foods that are useful for these stages will be discussed in the relevant sections in Part 3. What I describe here is a regime that will optimize your general health. Good nutrition is an excellent preventative.

**The basic logic behind this nutritional plan is:**

■ **Avoiding unnecessary strains on your body.** Foods that harm the body and challenge digestion, absorption or elimination will drain the body's energy reserve. Excess alcohol, for example, will not just evaporate into thin air – it will affect the lining of your gut, dehydrate your cells, trouble your liver, increase your heart rate and breathing, and affect your brain and the way you think. Similarly, too much coffee will tense your muscles, increase your heart rate, bring on muscle spasms, interfere with digestion, cause stress or irritability and reduce your body's healing power. Who needs such hassles from food? The net result is negative, not positive; pain, not pleasure. Choosing foods and drinks that put the body under minimal strain is a huge relief to all your systems.

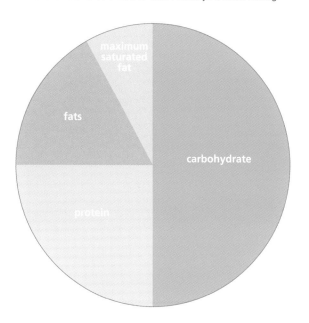

maximum saturated fat

fats

protein

carbohydrate

■ **Moderation.** Eating too much not only strains the digestive system, it will in time put pressure on vital organs such as the heart and liver. Eating too little, on the other hand, is likely to starve you of certain nutrients and may trigger your body into hoarding fat.

■ **A balance of all the essentials.** If something is lacking in the diet, the body's functions may be affected and the energy and the innate healing power will suffer. That will invariably lead to ill-health.

# Foods that are good for you

Whenever your body goes through hormonal changes – puberty, menstruation, pregnancy, the menopause – it is put under additional stress. The more stress your body experiences, the greater the need for vitamins, minerals and other micro-nutrients. There are certain nutrients that are especially pertinent to women.

## PROTEIN

An excess of animal protein usually goes hand in hand with excess saturated fat, with the associated problems of weight and heart or vascular disease. Too much animal protein has also been linked with osteoporosis. However, in my experience, women react to news like this by swinging too far the other way and start shunning protein. As always, it is a question of balance.

Too little protein can cause anaemia and low blood pressure, and contributes to fatigue, depression and often a poor immune system. The regular cycle of periodically building up and then shedding the lining of the womb creates a demand for protein, and crash dieters, vegans and anorexics, who starve themselves of protein, suffer water retention, scanty or irregular

periods, infertility and difficulties in pregnancy.

Protein provides us with amino acids, essential for our own protein synthesis, but only animal proteins and soya contain all eight essential amino acids. Strict vegetarians (who don't eat fish or eggs) therefore need to be aware of balancing their sources of proteins, rather than relying solely on grains and pulses.

Good sources of protein: To avoid the problem of eating too much fat-laden protein, choose predominantly fish and lean meats, and include plant proteins such as lentils, peas and beans; nuts, especially almonds, cashews, peanuts, and Brazil, hazel and pine nuts; mushrooms (but beware of fungus-based meat substitutes if you are intolerant of fungi); lower-fat cheeses such as cottage cheese, mozzarella or goat's cheese.

## VITAMINS AND MINERALS

### Vitamin D and calcium

Vitamin D helps us absorb calcium from food, vital for keeping teeth and bones strong. Calcium deficiency leads to problems with bones and joints and can cause osteoporosis. Although vitamin D is obtainable from only a limited number of sources, our requirements are modest and for most people there is little danger of a deficiency. These limited sources, however, put at risk anyone cut off from them, such as vegans and those who do not expose their skin to sunlight. Middle-aged and elderly Asian women are especially vulnerable. Many Asian women convert to veganism in their forties and fifties, restricting severely their protein intake at a time when they may need it the most, around the menopause. Later, they suffer badly from arthritis or backache, primarily caused by calcium deficiency.

Good sources: Vitamin D – oily fish, eggs, sunshine. Calcium – dairy foods, spinach, cabbage and kale, soya products, edible bones of oily fish such as sardines, many bottled waters.

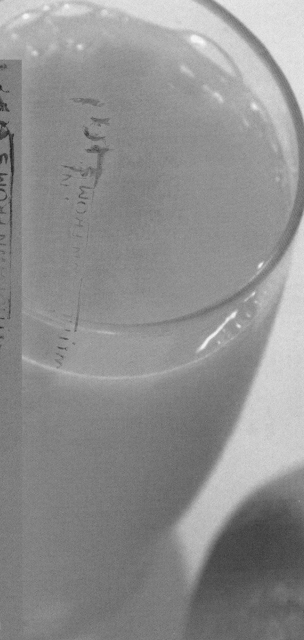

# FORTIFYING FOODSTUFFS

Some plants have properties that are particularly helpful in areas of concern to women.

- anaemia: spinach, aubergine, pomegranate, carrots, apples, cherries, lychees, sweeter varieties of clementines and tangerines, sugar cane, avocado, broccoli, beetroot. (NB the oxalates in spinach and beetroot can inhibit iron absorption, so boost your vitamin C at the same time with cabbage or sweet citrus fruits, to counteract)
- reproductive system: yam, rhubarb, pomegranate, ginger, saffron, cinnamon, chamomile, black cumin seeds (kolonji, Nigella sativa), coriander
- constipation: papaya, prunes, plums, okra, spinach, broccoli, asparagus, beetroot, melon, figs, salad leaves, cayenne pepper, chillis, sweet peppers, sweetcorn
- skin: turmeric, almonds, bitter gourd, carrots, pistachios, cardamom
- hair and nails: fish, marrow bone stock, aloe vera pulp, broccoli, pomegranate
- libido: yam, ginger, asafoetida, pistachios, raisins, eggs, nutmeg, saffron, black cumin seeds, ginseng
- mood enhancers: chamomile, ginger, dandelion tea, chicory, guarana, royal jelly, honey, mangoes (especially the sweeter variety with slight sour aftertaste, but also spiced mango chutney)

Always choose fruit and vegetables that have been well grown (look for organic labels or grow your own) and are as fresh as possible. If they have been grown in nutrient-deficient soil or had to travel long distances their nutritional content will be sadly lacking, even if they look good (waxing and preserving methods for long shelf-life do not help the nutrient content).

### Vitamin E

Fat-soluble Vitamin E is essential to the healthy functioning of the female reproductive system, helps keep skin healthy and wounds to heal well. Vitamin E is an antioxidant, which means it helps protect cells by 'mopping up' excess free radicals, unstable molecules that can harm our bodies.

Good sources: oily fish, wheatgerm oil, seeds and seed oils (sunflower, safflower), nuts, avocado.

### Vitamin B12

This vitamin is vital in the manufacture of blood, but the only people likely to suffer a deficiency are vegans (of which there are more women than men) because it is only available in animal products. Eggs and dairy produce will provide sufficient even if you don't eat meat or fish, but vegans may need to take a supplement.

### Folic acid (folate)

Normally, our ordinary diet will provide us with plenty of this B complex vitamin. However, it is recommended that you increase your intake significantly if you are planning to have a baby and during your pregnancy, as it provides protection against such congenital problems as spina bifida. You may need to take a supplement even if you eat plenty of the foods listed below.

Good sources: liver, brassicas such as cabbage and Brussels sprouts, spinach, eggs, peas.

### Iron

A major role of iron is in making the haemoglobin in blood, and too little leads to anaemia (anaemic blood actually looks less richly red). This is one of the few instances where the recommended requirement is higher for women than for men. Iron is lost during menstruation and many women are slightly anaemic some of the time.

Anaemia is particularly prevalent among teenage girls and during pregnancy. Vegetarians also need to check that they are getting enough iron. How well our bodies absorb iron is affected by other things we eat and drink – it is helped by vitamin C but impaired by, for example, caffeine and the oxalates in rhubarb and spinach.

Good sources: offal (especially liver), red meat, dried apricots, leafy green vegetables (the darker the better), eggs, soya meat-substitutes, seaweed, lentils, peas and beans, seeds and whole grains.

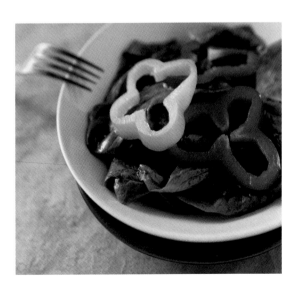

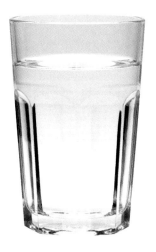
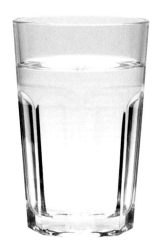
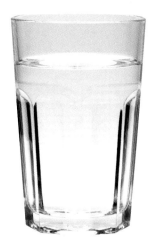
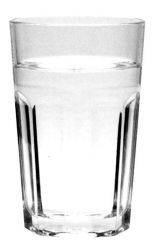
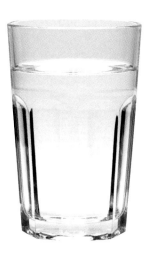

## WATER

Everyone is advised to drink about 1½ litres of water a day. Women who are concerned about water retention or abdominal bloating are inclined to restrict their fluid intake, thinking this will help. It doesn't.

Too little water can cause constipation, headaches, dry skin, bad body odour and halitosis, smelly urine, palpitations and sleep disturbances. Women are more badly affected by these last two, especially when they cause anxiety. And if this weren't enough, dehydration causes vaginal dryness, soreness of breasts (especially before periods) and water retention. Drinking more water also helps to flush through the urinary tract, which is more prone to infection in women than in men.

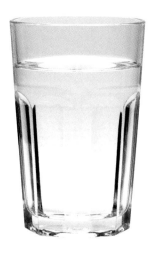
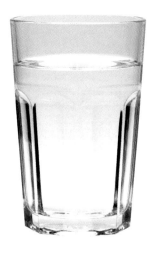
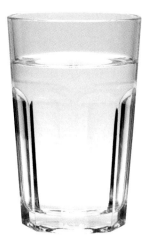

# Food and drink to avoid

Cutting out or keeping to a minimum certain types of food for at least four to six months will get your body functioning optimally, allowing it to regain its energy and restore its innate healing power. After that, if you have no problems, you may reintroduce some or all of them back into your diet in moderation, although many people find that after half a year of abstinence they no longer hanker after them, or even like them.

These restrictions are on …

◆ preserved products
◆ yeast
◆ sugar
◆ salt
◆ fatty foods
◆ caffeine
◆ alcohol

… and here's why.

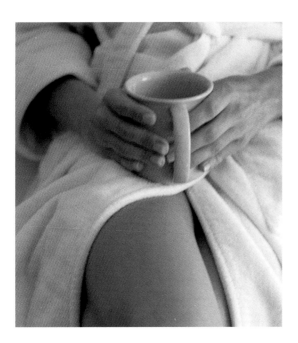

## STOMACH ACIDITY

A key point of the Lifestyle Programme is avoiding excess stomach acidity. This is the major cause of discordance in the digestive process. Many women experience uncomfortable upper abdominal bloating 30–45 minutes after eating as excess acid reacts with the bile and mucus is secreted by the small intestines, producing a lot of gas.

And indigestion, heartburn, stomach ulcers and other digestive complaints are not the only problems caused by acidity.

■ Stomach acid is the main stimulant of appetite, so it can be a contributory factor to weight problems.
■ Acidity affects collagen in the tendons, making them more prone to sports injuries and repetitive strain injuries, as well as making all sorts of everyday physical activities, from lifting babies to running up stairs, more difficult.
■ Chronic acidity can cause discoloration of the lips and mouth area, resulting in over-pink lips and the area around the mouth becoming pale and patchy (not as prominent as in vitiligo). I have known many women who have become concerned about their looks in this way but not understood its cause.
■ It is also possible that excess acid in the body can have a spermicidal effect, contributing to infertility.

For centuries, traditional physicians have considered citric and sour products bad for the body as they have been observed to increase the likelihood of:

◆ aches and pains around the body
◆ bruising
◆ skin rashes
◆ hair thinning
◆ teeth and gum problems, sour taste in the mouth, mouth ulcers, and cuts and abrasions on the side of the tongue

## WHY DOES EXCESS ACIDITY CAUSE SO MANY PROBLEMS?

**The digestive system is a fine balance of acid or alkaline media: the saliva in the mouth is alkaline, the gastric juices in the stomach are acidic and are then neutralized by bile, which is alkaline, in the small intestine. Bile is produced by the liver, but only in a limited amount each day. This is enough to cope with a regular balanced diet, but if what we eat and drink is extra-acidic, or if the stomach secretes excess acid, it will require a greater quantity of bile to neutralize it. This means that part-digested, highly acidic food can slow the digestive process and irritate the stomach walls, while waiting for the liver to produce more bile.**

◆ a slow-down in the healing process
◆ irritability
◆ bad breath and body odour
◆ stinging urine (even mimicking cystitis).

**Avoid:**

▧ citrus fruit and juices (e.g. orange, lemon, grapefruit)
▧ sour fruits and vegetables (e.g. pineapples, mangoes, kiwis, rhubarb, summer berries such as raspberries and strawberries, green apples, tamarind, tomatoes, passion fruit)
▧ vinegar, white wine and other acidic drinks
▧ canned sauces and pre-prepared meals (most include acidic preservatives) and vinegary pickled foods
▧ stomach irritants such as chilli, rich curries, nuts and seeds that have not been finely chewed or crushed, and over-hot beverages.

But the foods listed above are only part of the problem. Beware also of these other acid-producing factors:

▧ eating too fast. Food that is not chewed properly means more work for the stomach, which means it will have to produce more acidic gastric juice.
▧ smoking and recreational drugs.
▧ stress, which can lead to stomach ulcers and acidity. When the Russian physiologist Pavlov carried out his famous conditioned reflex experiments with dogs, he discovered that these animals under stress produced excess stomach acid and some even had ulcers.
▧ medicinal drugs when used over a prolonged period. Aspirin, anti-inflammatory drugs, steroids, strong doses of vitamin C (over 1,000 mg), and a host of drugs (from those used for chemotherapy and infertility to malaria tablets and antibiotics) cause acidity and even ulcers.
▧ bacterial infection, in particular Helicobacter pylori. This bacterium thrives in the stomach lining causing inflammation (gastritis) and ulcers.

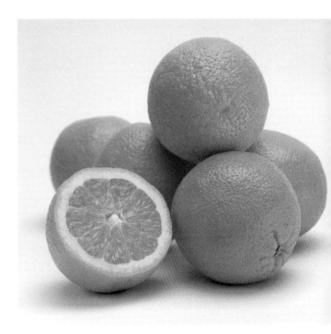

## PRESERVED PRODUCTS

The natural deterioration and rotting of food can be dramatically slowed by preservation. Commercially, this usually means adding chemical preservatives, salt, sugar and sometimes citric acid, to prevent bacterial or fungal growth.

Since a single can that has gone off will mean a recall of millions and a major loss to the manufacturer, food processors take no chances. Food and drink regulatory organizations have strict rules on the use of preservatives, but some manufacturers use minute doses of several chemical preservatives, which act synergistically to prevent bacterial or fungal growth. As each is below a level that needs to be declared on the label or that would attract the attention of our food and drink watchdogs, we are none the wiser.

Do not load your body with these chemicals, as, even though they pass through the regulatory bodies, they do not go unnoticed within our bodies. Skin, liver, stomach, kidneys are just some of the organs that may be affected.

### Avoid:
- food preserved in cans or cartons or commercially bottled.
- cured or preserved meat and fish. Even those not containing chemical preservatives will be very high in salt, sugar or vinegar, or all three.

## YEAST

Half a century ago, yeast, in the form of brewer's yeast, was a medicine and a good source of vitamin B. It was given to weak people, children and recuperating patients. It formed the essential component of most tonics. Today it causes a lot of harm to the body: it has become our enemy. What has caused this great change?

In nature there used to be a harmony among the three parasites that lived in our bodies: bacteria, viruses and fungi. Then in 1928 Sir Alexander Fleming discovered that a fungus, penicillium mould, was deadly to bacteria. In Fleming's time bacterial infection was a major cause of disease, and penicillin became the century's wonder drug, a revolution in medicine that would defeat the spread of bacteria. It worked extremely effectively and was viewed as the answer to every doctor's prayer. But bacteria are living entities and, to survive, they mutated and became resistant to this killer fungus. In response, antibiotics (for example, penicillin) were developed and by the 1960s were being widely but inappropriately used for all sorts of conditions. Bacterial resistance increased, and so began the escalation in the battle between man and bacteria – so that now we are facing threats from 'superbugs' such as MRSA. Meanwhile, opportunistic viruses and fungi took advantage of the weakened state of bacteria and, nowadays, viral and fungal infections dominate while bacterial infections are less common.

Yeast is a fungus that has easy access to the digestive system and other parts of the body. In a meshy parasitical variant called candida it sends out tentacle-like roots into vulnerable body tissue such as the mouth, intestines and vagina. It creates holes or patches in the normally impermeable gut walls, through which toxins pass into the bloodstream. Yeast also produces a toxic form of alcohol in the digestive system (see Sugar, below).

Candida and other bodily yeasts can trigger:
- bloating and gas
- vaginal thrush
- alopecia (bald patches on the scalp)
- skin rashes such as eczema and seborrhoeic dermatitis
- dandruff
- chronic fatigue
- weight gain (by increasing sugar cravings – glucose feeds candida).

Bile, produced by the liver, is a natural suppressant of candida growth in the digestive system, so anything that impairs the liver's function or overloads it can mean more freedom for candida. Alcohol and medical drugs, including the contraceptive pill and HRT, give the liver extra work to do.

**Avoid:**

- bread, including pizza and some flatbreads which contain yeast
- beer
- extract of yeast spread.

## SUGAR

Sugar is the favourite comfort food, but it is a false friend. In excess it is a major contributor to:

- weight gain
- chronic fatigue
- skin problems (eczema, psoriasis)
- mood swings (particularly premenstrually)
- abdominal gas.

Not only is sugar fattening, it is also very hard to give up. Because it is quickly assimilated into the system, it gives an instant relief to hunger pangs, a quick burst of energy and a psychological 'lift'. However, the effect is fleeting, and hunger, fatigue or a sense of lowness soon return, stronger than before. Where there is an emotional problem, sugary foods form the basis of binge-eating, resulting in waves of highs and lows that are difficult to cope with.

And sugar has another effect on the body. As explained above, our bodies are more prone than they used to be to harbouring yeasts, and yeast + sugar + warmth + time = alcohol. Excess sugar will encourage fermentation in a sluggish digestion system, so that even though you may not be drinking alcohol regularly, you could be producing your own 'hooch', which of course is not as controlled as a commercial brewery. This can have toxic effects on the liver and the rest of your body. Bloating and rumbling of the tummy is an indication of this type of gut fermentation, as is fatigue after eating.

## SALT

Some of the long-term complications of consuming too much salt include:

- water retention
- high blood pressure
- anxiety or irritability
- increased tendency to aches and pains (period pains may get worse)
- worse PMS.

Particular care has to be taken to restrict salt intake during pregnancy, when excess salt poses a risk of pre-eclampsia and eclampsia, serious complications of pregnancy and a danger to the mother and the unborn baby (see page 169).

## FATTY FOODS

Butter, cream, cheese, fried and oily food, the fat in meat such as pork, lamb and beef all add to your stores of body fat. As well as causing weight problems, these heavy, solid fats, known as saturated fats, also:

- put a strain on the digestive system, which leads to further health problems
- raise cholesterol levels, clogging arteries and leading to heart and vascular disease to a level that becomes life-threatening.

Consume fewer fats, replace butter in cooking with vegetable or seed oil and cream by low-fat yoghurt, and your skin will be healthier, your body lighter, your joints more mobile and your mind clearer.

## CAFFEINE

All over the world, humans have exploited plant extracts that give a rush of short-term euphoria or alter the consciousness in some way – marijuana, mezcal, Polynesian kava, opium. Caffeine is also a stimulant, but coffee has become an integral part of society, from the tiny cardamom-scented cupful with which an Arab shopkeeper might greet you, to a ritual morning espresso in an Italian café. The resurgence of coffee shops provides office workers from Seattle to Swindon with frothy cappuccinos without which they feel they cannot start the day. In these days of heightened 'alcohol awareness', coffee shops have become the new bars.

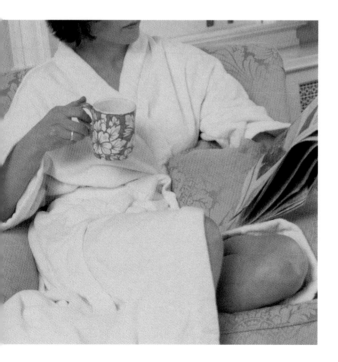

Over 200 years ago, Samuel Hahneman, the founder of homeopathy, said that coffee was the worst thing we could consume. Like other stimulants or suppressants, coffee is addictive and it is regular drinking that brings trouble – stop suddenly and you get withdrawal symptoms such as headaches and anxiety attacks. Such a thing cannot be good.

Caffeine affects the body by:

- increasing heart and breathing rate
- tensing muscles
- constricting blood vessels, reducing oxygen supply to the tissues
- raising metabolic rate and blood pressure
- causing gas formation and irritation in the gut (so should definitely be avoided by those who have irritable bowels)
- causing dehydration.

Most of these symptoms mimic the panicky feeling of stress, and eat into the body's energy system by forcing everything to race. This is especially bad news at times when it is most helpful to keep your body calm, such as before and during periods, while trying to conceive, while pregnant or breastfeeding, and during the menopause. It also makes emotions harder to control.

Coffee, being a diuretic, increases urine secretion, and the increased sweating from the racing of the heart also releases more fluid from your body. This dehydration can slow down the body's functions. In traditional coffee-drinking countries, a cup of coffee is accompanied by a glass of water, to counteract its diuretic effect.

Women who are regular coffee-drinkers often get benign hardening in the breasts, causing tenderness especially before periods. Too much coffee can also increase period pains and constrict the Fallopian tubes, affecting fertility. I have found that women who have given up coffee have reported that their symptoms improve dramatically.

## ALCOHOL

Nowadays, women drink almost as much alcohol as men do; it has become part of social life and alcoholism among women is increasing worryingly. Binge drinking and frequent drunkenness are not only a direct threat to women's health, but lay them open to abuse and 'date rape' drugs.

Most people know that chronic alcohol abuse damages the liver by scarring or cirrhosis (hardening) as the liver cells are deprived of oxygen. Overloading the liver can have other side-effects, though, some of which are particularly relevant to women:

■ Because the liver manufactures most of the clotting factors of the blood, liver damage may lead to a tendency to haemorrhage, making periods long and unusually heavy.

■ This same tendency to haemorrhage can cause easy and unsightly bruising.

■ The contraceptive pill or HRT put the liver under strain (read the small print under side-effects), so alcohol becomes an additional burden on an already hard-worked organ.

It has been found that women have a lower tolerance to alcohol than men, so are more easily and quickly afflicted by the problems that beset all who drink too much:

◆ drying and premature ageing of the skin, accompanied by reddening of nose and cheeks from broken blood vessels
◆ other unattractive features, such as bad breath, bloodshot eyes and dandruff
◆ tremors in the hands

## A FINAL ITEM TO AVOID

Smoking. Pregnant women and those around babies and young children are always advised not to smoke, but what about women themselves?

Despite many years of medical advice, media campaigning and education in schools, young people, and girls at an even greater rate than boys, continue to take up smoking. Peer pressure and wanting to appear adult and 'cool' are undoubtedly powerful motives, but among girls there is also a misconception that smoking helps to keep you thin. There is no substance to this (see page 223).

Nicotine does bring a temporary sense of relaxation as it dilates the blood vessels, but this small benefit is far outweighed by the risks, lung cancer and other respiratory diseases, long-term complications in the heart and smaller blood vessels, to name just a few. It is also more addictive than many illegal drugs associated with addiction.

◆ fluid retention (causing bloating)
◆ short-term memory loss
◆ loss of libido
◆ poor sleep pattern and increased irritability (alcohol induces sleep, but its dehydrating effect will wake you prematurely)
◆ addiction.

My advice is to drink only occasionally and moderately, with particular awareness of any familial cases of alcoholism and your own state of health. Women generally avoid alcohol during pregnancy and while breastfeeding. It is also best to avoid it also while trying to conceive and just before and during periods: alcohol exacerbates PMS.

# Exploring the pleasures of food

Nutrition is not simply a matter of following a list of dos and don'ts: eating should be a positive part of life, not a guilty pleasure or a reluctant adherence to rules you are constantly longing to break. Establish a good relationship with food and healthy eating will become the norm.

## Eat with all your senses

Let all your senses enjoy the food you eat: how it looks, how it smells, how it feels on the tongue. Learn to discern different flavours. Eating slowly will allow you to savour food to the full and also put a natural brake on eating too much – stop when you think that another mouthful will fill you up.

## Cook

Preparing meals yourself will ensure you know what has gone into the food on your plate. You will have greater control over your own and your family's eating habits. Get involved in shopping for food, as it will create the fundamentals of a healthy diet. If you avoid buying foods that you are know are not healthy, then nobody will have the opportunity to eat bad things. Try out different recipes and encourage all the family to learn to cook. Make eating out an occasional treat, rather than relying on takeaways or fast food as regular standbys.

## Add variety

The basic tastes are sweet, sour, bitter, salty, pungent (spicy) and astringent. (A seventh, often added, is insipid, as in water.) The Chinese try to include all of these in a meal, and aiming for this kind of variety will avoid the dangers that boredom brings. Even bitter, so often disliked, has its place, as it sharpens up all other tastes – if you did not have darkness, you could never enjoy the light. Two to three tastes on the one plate is ideal, I feel, to bring variety without overloading the tastebuds.

Much of the flavour and interest in our meals comes from fats, salt, sugar, herbs or spices. You can devise a nutritionally perfect eating regime, but if it is bland it will be boring, and soon have you craving for stimulating flavour – which probably means reaching for something fatty, salty or sweet.

To avoid falling into this trap, experiment with different herbs and spices. There are so many to choose from. Use chillies and strong spices in moderation, as when overdone they produce excess stomach acid (especially when fried in oil).

## Fast

Fasting from time to time or on a regular basis will make sure that your digestive system and your liver and kidneys get a rest. It also helps keep weight in check and reinforces the will to keep to a healthy diet. In India, unless they are pregnant or during their periods, women fast or semi-fast at least once a week, eating one simple meal a day and avoiding any grains.

Try fasting or semi-fasting regularly once a week – this is especially beneficial for anyone with weight or digestive problems. For more on how to undertake a regular or occasional fast, see page 230.

## THE BENEFITS OF FASTING

- helping weight loss
- de-stressing your body, improving sleep and lightening mood
- resting your liver, which has to detoxify everything you eat and drink
- allowing your digestive system to rest and carry out any necessary regenerative work
- enhancing your body's innate healing power to combat disease and illness
- reinforcing your willpower

## Eating by the Lifestyle

How do all these principles translate into everyday eating?
The following is not a meal plan to follow like a dietary
prescription, but aims to show you how the theory can be
applied in practice – you will have your own preferences,
and quite possibly a partner or family to take into
account. These guidelines should also be useful when
choosing from a menu when you are eating out.

### BREAKFAST

**Choose:**

- cereals: wholegrain or porridge, rather than
  processed or sweetened
- fruit: whole fruit are better than just juices,
  especially acidic citrus juices
- yoghurt
- eggs: boiled or poached rather than fried (or
  scramble in a non-stick saucepan)
- bread/toast: try soda bread (which is yeast-free),
  crispbreads, matzos or oatcakes instead of regular
  bread
- spreads: honey rather than jams, marmalade or
  salty processed spreads – and limit your butter too
- tea, rather than coffee

**Avoid:**

- traditional 'full English' fried breakfast
- orange/grapefruit juice
- sweet or buttery pastries (croissants, Danish pastries,
  etc.)
- coffee

### MAIN MEALS (LUNCH OR DINNER)

**Choose:**

- fish
- chicken breast
- mixed salads
- mixed or basmati rice
- new potatoes
- grilled vegetables

  followed by fruit salad

**Avoid:**

- fatty cuts of meat or sausages
- rich curries or very hot dishes
- chips or creamy mash
- cream sauces and rich dressings

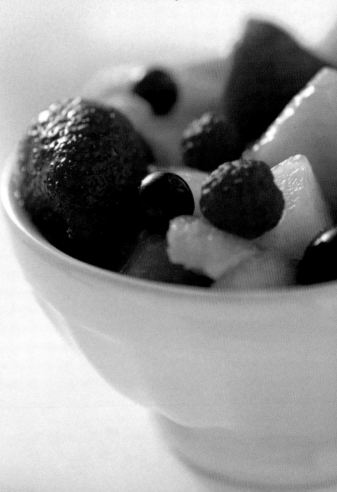

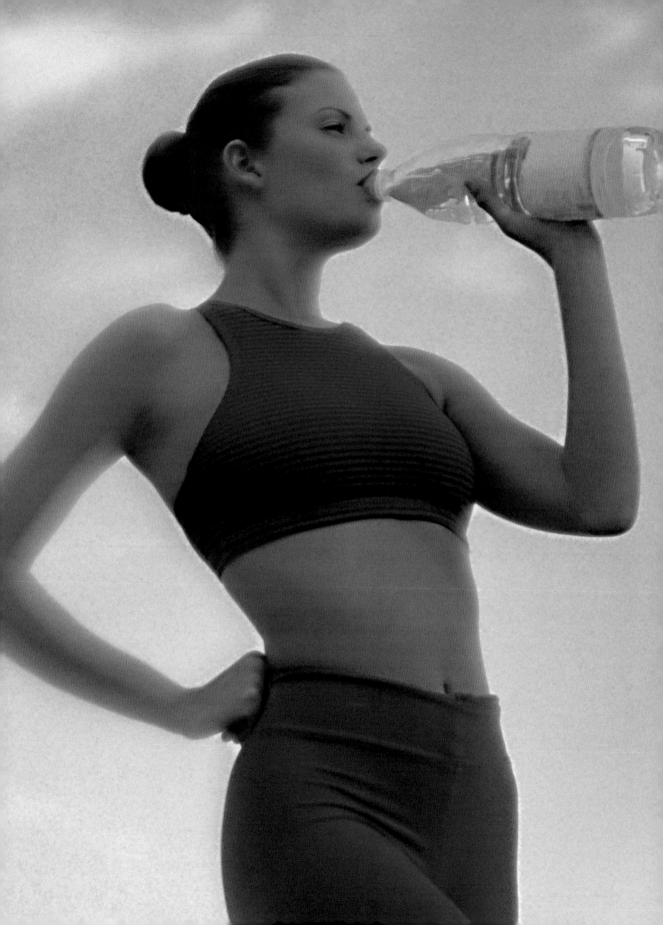

## HOME-MADE CHICKEN SOUP

**This highly nutritious broth makes a great sustaining food in all sorts of circumstances: to restore energy after childbirth, when you are ill and have no appetite, if you have digestive problems or whenever you are feeling run down.**

**Chop a poussin or young organic chicken and crush the leg and thigh bones. Add to a pan with 2½–3 litres of water with ginger, garlic, bay leaves, cinnamon, cardamom pods and a pinch of turmeric. Bring to the boil and simmer for an hour. Strain. Drink this stock two or three times a day. You can also use it as a base for a soup.**

### EXTRAS

Snacks are useful on days when there is an unavoidably long gap between meals, and many people find they operate better on several small meals a day. But don't snack instead of eating proper meals, or out of boredom or frustration.

#### Choose:

- fresh or dried (not candied) fruit
- smoothies
- ready-prepared vegetables, such as carrot batons or celery sticks
- mini-pitta breads with dips such as hummus or guacamole
- yoghurt
- nuts (chestnuts are the lowest in fat; unsalted peanuts and cashews are lower than Brazils, pecans or hazelnuts)
- seeds, such as pumpkin, sesame or sunflower

#### Avoid:

- sweets and chocolate bars
- crisps and extruded food products
- cakes and sweet biscuits

### DRINKS

#### Choose:

- water
- apple, grape, blackcurrant, cranberry juices rather than citrus juices. Ideally, squeeze your own, but if buying in a bottle or carton, ensure it is 100 per cent juice and not 'juice drink' or just labelled to look like pure juice
- tea, especially herbal teas
- milk with a little honey at bedtime

#### Avoid:

- coffee
- alcohol
- sugary squashes
- citrus or sour juices
- fizzy drinks

## TEAS AND TISANES

**Teas and tisanes can be useful for different times of the day:**

**Morning – dandelion, chicory**
**During the day – ginseng**
**Evening – chamomile, rose**

**Massage** has always held a powerful therapeutic value. More than just a benefit for circulation, massage can produce maximum energy in the muscles, and muscles kept toned and well nourished will be full of energy.

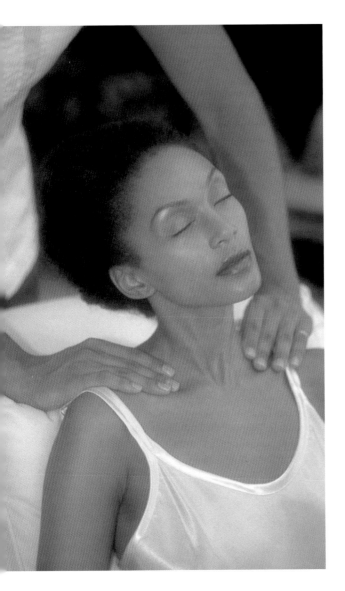

Until comparatively recently, the standard form of massage in the Western world was based on the gentle rotatory Swedish massage, which is still the most widespread. All European massage schools teach to 'massage towards the heart' with the idea of improving blood circulation.

Traditional eastern massage, on the other hand, massages in both directions but mainly away from the heart, focusing on the muscles, joints, ligaments, tendons and skin. Such massage is anatomically and therapeutically more precise. Alternately squeezing and relieving the pressure on the muscles moves lactic acid into the bloodstream where it can be broken down by oxygen more quickly.

## The vital role played by the neck

Neck and shoulder massage forms an important part of my technique. The topmost, or cervical, vertebrae that make up the neck form protective canals through which run a pair of arteries known as the vertebral arteries. They are the best-protected arteries in the entire body because they are crucial to our existence. They supply blood to the subconscious brain, the older part of our brain, evolutionarily speaking, which is responsible for everything that might be considered automatic, from breathing to fluid balance.

But these cervical vertebrae are highly mobile and vulnerable. Whiplash injuries, jarring falls, bumps to the head, contact sports, hours spent at the computer screen, drawing board or desk, long-haul flights, even high pillows – these all put strain on the neck and can cause dislocation or misalignment of these delicate bones. Twisting or distortion can also happen during birth, and cranial osteopathy can be very helpful in subtly adjusting the alignment in a young baby (see page 182).

Once that happens, the vertebral canal loses its uniformity and can constrict the blood vessels inside. This leads to impaired functions of one or the other regulatory nerve centres of the subconscious brain. Here are some examples.

## ENERGY

A reduced blood supply to the subconscious brain means a reduced oxygen and glucose supply. Chronic fatigue sets in. As the brain feels 'starved', it sends signals for food, particularly glucose. This leads to sugar cravings, which in turn can lead to weight problems or hyperactivity.

## SLEEP

Problems with the brain's sleep centre typically result in a jet-lag type of sleep pattern – alert at night, tired during the day. This is because the secretion of melatonin has been affected. Melatonin is often called a 'rejuvenating' hormone as it maintains the restful state of the body, allowing the body to repair damage and injuries. When the day/night wake/sleep rhythm is upset it has all sorts of repercussions beyond tiredness, including:

- mood swings
- depression
- headaches
- loss of concentration

- hormonal disturbance
- reduced daytime performance.

Each day becomes a struggle to get through.

## HORMONAL BALANCE

The area fed by the vertebral arteries includes the pituitary gland, which controls most of our hormones. If the pituitary or its companion gland, the hypothalamus, malfunctions it can result in thyroid problems (weight gain and fatigue), ovarian problems (polycystic ovaries, perhaps endometriosis, infertility, poor or irregular periods), adrenal problems (cellulite, weight gain) or fluid retention (under the control of the hypothalamus).

# The subconscious brain at its optimum

The pituitary and hypothalamus together regulate a wide range of our automatic functions, including heartbeat, breathing, digestion, appetite and energy levels, immune system, hormone regulation, emotions, sleep, fluid retention, body temperature control and libido.

Using my technique of neck massage helps these all-important parts of the brain function better and alleviates a wide range of conditions. Here are some examples.

## REGULATING THE IMMUNE SYSTEM

The pituitary gland, together with the adrenal glands, regulates the immune system. More women than men suffer from auto-immune diseases such as lupus, rheumatoid arthritis, Raynaud's syndrome and Crohn's disease. I have treated these conditions with my neck massage technique, which gently adjusts the vertebrae and reduces tension in the muscles and tendons that tighten that area. The results are quicker than, for example, cranial osteopathy, and definitely long lasting, as the blood is able to carry more oxygen and glucose to the brain than cerebrospinal fluid can. Although the results can only be anecdotal in scientific terms, they are very satisfactory when it comes to the number of patients who have been helped.

Since neck stiffness is a common symptom of stress, it may also be that the onset of diseases that have a link to stress (which can range from cancer to psoriasis) may be connected to a weakening of the immune system.

## REGULATING HORMONES

The pituitary and hypothalamus regulate several hormones of importance to women:

◆ **oxytocin** causes contractions in the uterus during labour
◆ **prolactin** develops breast tissue and helps the glands to secrete more milk, while suppressing ovulation and periods
◆ **growth hormones**, when they are under- or overworking, can lead to great self-consciousness and psychological problems
◆ **androgens/oestrogens**, the male and female hormones respectively, are present in both women and men but in very different proportions. An imbalance in one or the other has implications for a woman's normal development and reproductive ability, and can also be responsible for conditions as varied as cellulite and excess body hair.

A well-regulated hormonal flow can help the body with all aspects of reproduction and pregnancy – this is covered in more detail in Part 3.

## BALANCING THE EMOTIONS

Just behind the hypothalamus and slightly above it is an area of the brain known as the limbic system. Here lie nerve centres that control a wide variety of elements of our existence, from waking and sleeping to sexual drive and the control of emotions. Panic attacks, depression, mood swings, post-natal depression and other emotional turmoils are strongly linked to this area of the brain.

Women are often described as multi-tasking, taking on a wide range of different tasks and roles – wife, mother, housewife, family welfare manager, breadwinner, social organizer – which call up a wide range of emotions. Coping with these successfully depends on the proper functioning of the limbic system, which relies on the optimal circulation of cerebral fluid and blood to the brain. In my opinion, all women need neck, shoulder and even head massages on a regular basis, to help them with the emotional demands and drain on energy of a roller-coaster life.

Massage as a way of treating some of these conditions may sound odd, and most doctors would not believe its therapeutic effects. However, years of trials and observations mean that I have time and time again seen the efficacy of treatment by therapeutic massage.

# The basic moves

Although only trained therapists with a good knowledge of the anatomy of the skull, neck, shoulder and back can carry out this therapy in full, self-help can be beneficial.

Do the following massage routine perhaps twice a week, either at bedtime, or while you are in the shower or bath (with oil). Even better, involve a partner; it is easier to massage someone else rather than yourself, and you will both have the pleasure and benefit of this wonderful but absolutely necessary treatment.

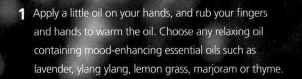

1 Apply a little oil on your hands, and rub your fingers and hands to warm the oil. Choose any relaxing oil containing mood-enhancing essential oils such as lavender, ylang ylang, lemon grass, marjoram or thyme.

2 Place the tips of the fingers on the ear lobes and slide your hands down to reach the top of the neck. From here down to the shoulders, massage the sides of the neck using your fingers and thumbs in a rotatory movement. The bony lumps you can feel are the lateral projections of the seven vertebrae of the cervical spine. Some of these hard points will feel sore. Massage gently at first and increase pressure as tolerance develops. The vertebral arteries are located deep within these vertebrae, and gentle movements and vibrations help to loosen them up and ultimately facilitate the blood flow.

3 After 2–3 minutes, move your fingers a little inwards, towards the central axis of the back. Now you will feel taut 'strings' of muscles and tendons of the neck. Massage these, working up and down the neck. Some muscles and tendons will be sore.

4 Next, grab the top of the shoulder (the bulk of the trapezius muscles), and alternately squeeze and release to encourage blood circulation. You may feel some lumps or knots, caused by spasms of muscles due to lactic acid or nerve irritation in the neck. Rub these with extra vigour, kneading with your thumbs.

5 Use your fingers and thumbs to reach the back of the skull (the occiput), just above the hairline. This is where the tendons of the neck muscles attach, and when the neck muscles are tense, these tendons are quite sore. As you work, the tenderness will ease and feel better.

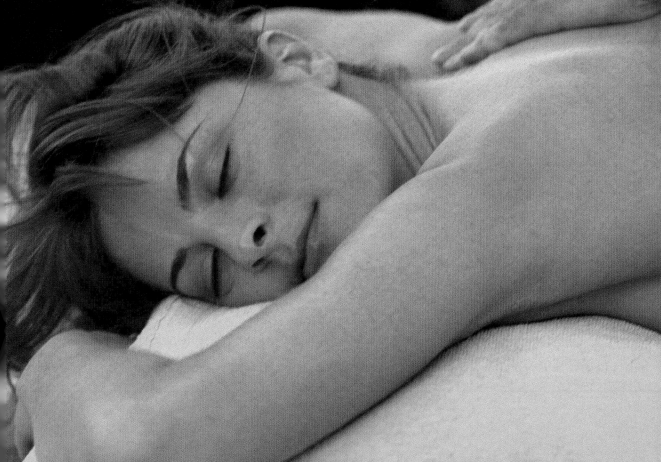

# Exercise stimulates and strengthens the muscles, joints, tendons, heart, lymphatic and nervous systems and the circulation, helping to renew blood supply to the tissues and remove waste products.

Many different forms of exercise have a valuable role, but I particularly recommend yoga because of its powerful therapeutic value.

## The benefits of yoga

Yoga is a marvellous antidote to the physical and emotional stresses women are subjected to in their daily lives. Yoga:

- increases flexibility
- builds up strength without overdeveloping the muscles
- improves blood flow to the brain, in particular the subconscious brain
- instils discipline and patience
- stills the mind
- has a calming and invigorating effect.

Many forms of exercise, especially competitive sports, can lead to injuries as the competitive element overrules the body's own flexibility and limits of endurance. Yoga is extremely unlikely to cause any harm, especially if done under a qualified and experienced teacher. The health-giving powers of yoga are explored in more detail in my book *Therapeutic Yoga* (Vermilion 2002).

Although vigorous variations of yoga have their own 'kick', the real feel-good factor comes from the slow and steady rhythm of hatha yoga combined with pranayama (breathing). Controlled breathing is highly therapeutic, the most powerful communication with the subconscious brain.

On pages 76–81 you will find a special section on Living Yoga. This is an adaptation of a wonderfully practical series of exercises by a yoga master, that I have modified to suit a modern working woman, so they can be tailored to your own routine. Incorporating these exercises into your daily routine in this way also provides a regular gentle reminder to care for your health, emotions and well-being.

In addition to the general routine and asanas (postures) described in Living Yoga, you will find specific moves in Part 3 that are particularly efficacious for certain conditions or circumstances.

## Other forms of exercise

The types of exercise suggested in the chapter on Weight Control – swimming, dancing, walking and tai chi – are particularly good if you are overweight, but they are excellent exercise for everyone at every age.

When incorporating more physical exercise into your life, choose something that suits your lifestyle and appeals to you. If you force yourself to go to the gym even though you hate it, you will end up finding excuses not to go. If you take up swimming even though ferrying the children to a child-minder, getting to a pool and

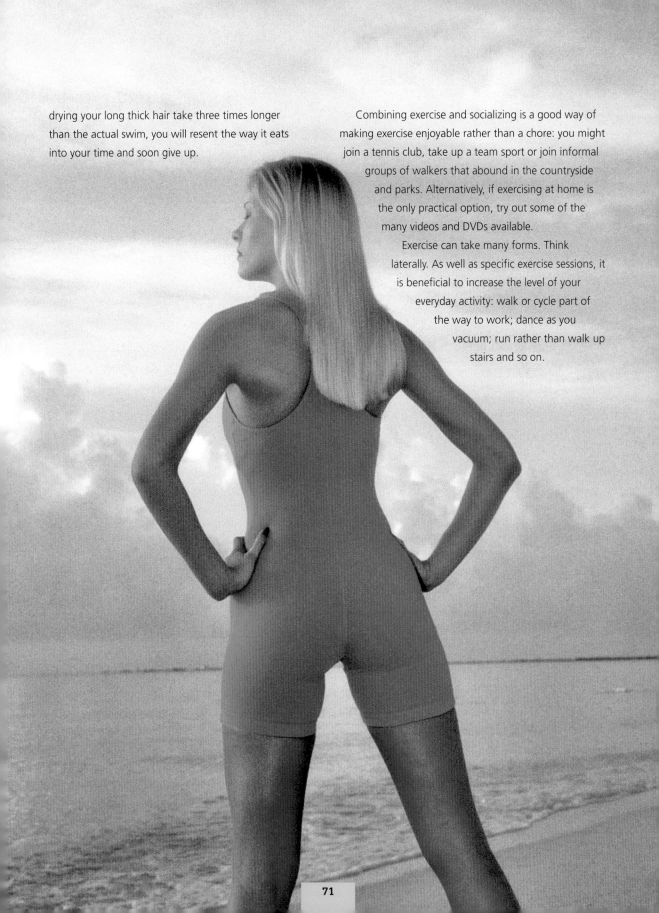

drying your long thick hair take three times longer than the actual swim, you will resent the way it eats into your time and soon give up.

Combining exercise and socializing is a good way of making exercise enjoyable rather than a chore: you might join a tennis club, take up a team sport or join informal groups of walkers that abound in the countryside and parks. Alternatively, if exercising at home is the only practical option, try out some of the many videos and DVDs available.

Exercise can take many forms. Think laterally. As well as specific exercise sessions, it is beneficial to increase the level of your everyday activity: walk or cycle part of the way to work; dance as you vacuum; run rather than walk up stairs and so on.

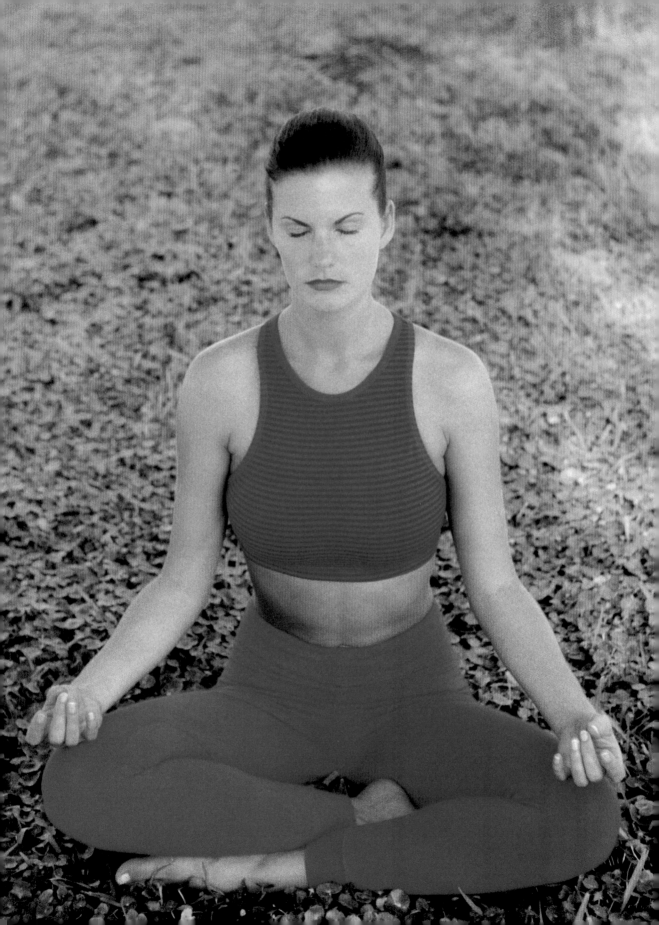

# Relaxation

In this age of high stress, with pressures at work and at home and demanding lives that leave no space to just 'be', there is a demand for relaxation. And the mind needs rest, just as the body does.

You can use a variety of methods to still your mind: chanting, praying, contemplation, concentration, auto-suggestion, meditation, visualization and yoga are all good disciplines. I have opted for relaxation through controlled breathing because it gives quicker results and is very practical. As our muscles relax, there is less resistance to the flow of blood so general circulation improves. Relaxed muscles reduce pressure on the brain (tranquillizers and sedatives work on the brain, reducing tension in the body as a whole) and this induces sleep by calming the mind. Through controlling your breathing you learn to control your subconscious mind.

To get into the habit, set aside the same time every day. A good suggestion is at the end of the working day, when 20 minutes of following this relaxation technique will help you to unwind, and provide a break between your working life and your domestic and social life in the evenings. It is a habit worth forming. You will not only feel more relaxed, revived and re-energized but, done regularly, this simple form of relaxation will help to lower blood pressure, reduce stress levels and improve concentration.

## The technique

Lie still on your back on the bed, or on the floor cushioned with blankets so you are comfortable. Rest your arms by your side, close your eyes and then begin to breathe as described overleaf for retention breathing.

## Controlled breathing

There is more than one way of breathing:

- **upper chest breathing:** very shallow and short, failing to aerate the entire lungs. The neck muscles lift the ribcage a little and the diaphragm moves minimally.

- **chest breathing:** when the muscles connecting the ribs contract, the ribcage expands rather like a folded umbrella being opened; it then contracts when the muscles relax.

- **diaphragmal breathing:** here, the diaphragm flattens and increases the volume of the chest cavity.

- **abdominal:** the most advanced and deepest form of breathing. The abdominal wall bellows out when breathing in and the diaphragm flattens as the air rushes in. When exhaling the abdominal wall is sucked in, pushing the diaphragm up, expelling as much air out of the lungs as possible.

I advocate this fourth type. Deeper breathing and breath retention improve oxygen uptake. While you are holding your breath and exhaling, the body retains carbon dioxide in the blood, which is then exchanged for oxygen in the next inhalation. A fascinating thing is that it is exchanged molecule for molecule with carbon dioxide –

so the more carbon dioxide you retain in the blood, the more oxygen you get in return. The slower you breathe, the more oxygen you get. Exactly the opposite happens during a panic attack, sexual intercourse or physical exercise: rapid, shallow breathing fails to supply sufficient oxygen and the mind and the body get more excited. The slower you breathe, the calmer you are.

Activating the diaphragm massages the internal organs and improves blood circulation to them.

The following are basic breathing exercises that can be done at any time, and are often referred to in part 3.

## Exercise 1

◼ Breathe in and out to a normal rhythm, but bellow your abdomen out as you breathe in and exhale by sucking the abdomen right in.

◼ Pushing your abdomen out during inhalation and sucking it in during exhalation is exactly the opposite of what most people do. While bellowed out, the abdomen creates negative pressure in the abdominal cavity and so the diaphragm flattens out and moves downwards, and blood rushes to the abdomen from the lower part of the body. When the abdomen is sucked in, the diaphragm domes and blood is pushed up towards the heart.

## Exercise 2

◼ Quick in-out-in-out breaths (expanding and contracting your abdomen as before) helps to exchange air efficiently.

## Exercise 3 (retention breathing)

Lie comfortably on your back. Breathe in for 3 seconds (abdomen out), hold your breath for 3 seconds (with practice, you can prolong this to 6 seconds) and breathe out (abdomen in) over 6 seconds.

◼ Breathing slowly and alternating the expansion and contraction of your abdomen correctly requires a bit of practice, but once you have mastered this it is a powerful method of stress relief and relaxation.

You may initially feel lightheaded and even panicky as your anxious and fatigued mind and body are demanding oxygen and you are restricting it. But as the oxygen supply to your body increases, your brain (whose main fuel is glucose and oxygen) benefits and, as you relax, it gets energized.

Once your breathing is controlled, divert your thoughts to different parts of your body, focusing on each area for three to five seconds, in the following sequence:

◼ **Cycle 1:** forehead—eyebrows—top of your head—temples—back of your head—neck—shoulders—upper back—mid-back—lower back—thighs—calves—ankles—feet—toes.

◼ **Cycle 2:** forehead—eyebrows—top of your head—temples—back of your head—neck—shoulders—upper arms—forearms—hands—fingertips.

Repeat each cycle three times.

Continue the slow, deep breathing. Your entire body will feel relaxed and heavy. Concentrate on your nostrils as you breathe. Cool air goes in and warm air goes out. Focus on this sensation for a minute or so. Relax your jaw, your throat and then your heart. Imagine that the heart is slowing down.

You may drift into deep sleep. When you wake up, begin to breathe as before for a few cycles. Move your toes. Move your fingers and slowly open your eyes to absorb the world again. You must follow this last step or you can become self-hypnotized and go into a trance. Use your thoughts to move each part of your body again.

Get up slowly. Have a drink of water or a cup of tea.

## Moderation  The body and the mind are designed to deal with a certain level of work and stress at a time.

The digestive system cannot cope with a regular overload of heavy food, and starving yourself forces your body to take defensive action by going into famine mode, shutting down systems to survive. Muscles and joints under constant strain will develop RSI (repetitive strain injury), while those that are never moved will stiffen up or atrophy. Life is a matter of balance. If you have been putting too many demands on your body, you need to allow it compensatory rest: sleep after too much action, fasting after too much food. An alternative, perhaps more practical, approach is to practise moderation.

In the Nutrition section (see pages 51–65), for example, I describe the foods that cause maximum harm. Unless you have an allergy, these foods won't individually cause much trouble – problems arise with an excess. If you overload your digestive system with pizza, cheese, chillies, nuts, orange juice, creamy cake, coffee and brandy all at once, your body will revolt. Instead, play a balancing game. If you have drunk coffee then perhaps pass on alcohol that day; if you have had too much bread, perhaps eat fewer citrus fruits. Respect your body and don't overtax it.

It is generally good advice that if you avoid what is most harmful to the body, it will cope better with what is less harmful. The body has a tremendous capacity to adapt itself and that is the true gift of nature. If you minimize what is potentially harmful and eat sensibly, exercise regularly but without reaching straining point, balance the busyness of your life with times of quiet, you will sustain health and well-being.

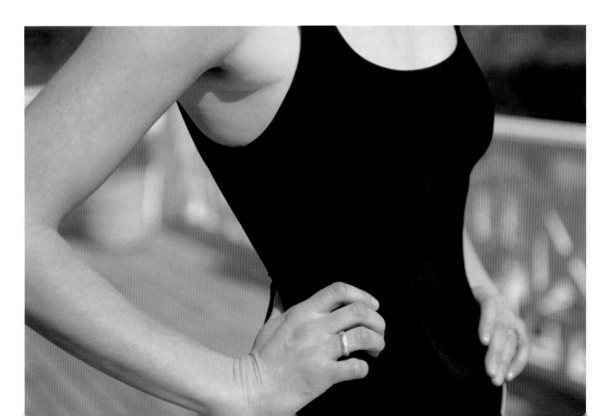

# Living yoga through the day   This is a terrific daily routine based on Living Yoga developed by my 90-year-old yoga master, Air Vice-Marshal Suren Goel MBE.

Finding a complete hour to do exercises is often difficult when you have a busy schedule, so what he suggests is a series of yogic and other short exercises that can be done through the day as a minute here and a minute there. This makes it a perfect form of exercise easily adopted in today's busy world. At first you may need to keep reminding yourself about even so simple a routine, but soon it will be as habitual as brushing your teeth.

## ON WAKING

You have just woken up, your eyes feel heavy and you might want to sleep a bit longer. You still feel lethargic. While lying on your back:

1  Rub your eyes gently with your fingers.
2  Squeeze and release your eyebrow area with your thumb and index finger.
3  With your thumb gently massage above the bridge of your nose and in the innermost corner of your eye sockets.
4  With all your fingers, massage your jaws (they might be slightly sore).
5  Squeeze and release your ear lobes and work upwards, squeezing all parts of your ear.
6  Massage the sides of your neck. Squeeze and release the back of your neck with your hands.
7  Massage your scalp with your fingertips and thumbs by moving your skin over your skull rather than moving your fingers against your skin. Work your way all over your scalp.

8  Massage your temples with your fingers (these might feel sore).
9  Place your arms by your sides. Take a deep breath, bellowing out your abdomen as you do so. Hold your breath to the count of three, then suck in your abdomen as you very slowly breathe out fully. Repeat 10 times.
10  Bend your knees, with your feet flat on the bed, keeping your ankles and feet hip-distance apart. Take a deep breath in, bellowing out your abdomen as before, and raise your pelvis as high as you can. Draw your chin closer to your chest. Hold your breath while you count to five. You'll feel the blood rushing to your face and head. Slowly let yourself back down, starting with your upper back and sequentially going down to let your buttocks touch last. Stretch the spine towards your legs as you do so: this releases the tension in the lower back by extending the spine. Breathe out slowly during this descent, sucking in your abdomen to empty the lungs effectively. Repeat five times.
You are now wide awake.

## IN THE BATHROOM

If you don't have the urge to empty your bowels, drink a couple of glasses of water and massage your abdomen clockwise with your hands five times. This should encourage your bowels into action.

After brushing your teeth, gargle with lukewarm water and massage your gums for a minute or so.

If possible fit in 10 minutes of yoga exercises. The salutation to the sun (see overleaf) is a complete exercise form.

When showering, massage your body vigorously; this helps tone up the muscles for the day. In particular, massage:

◆ the sides of your neck, squeezing across your shoulders.

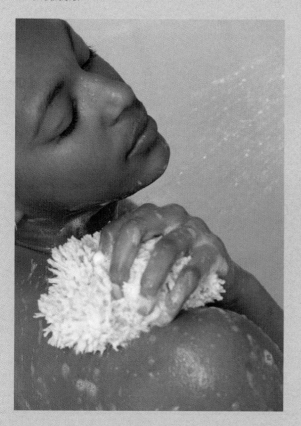

◆ your arms from the shoulder right down to the wrist. Concentrate especially on the extensors and flexors of your lower arm if you are going to be at a computer for much of the day.

◆ each hand with your thumbs, focusing on the area at the base of the thumb. This helps to prevent RSI.

◆ your buttocks (they get tired if you are sitting all day at a desk), thighs and calves.

Allowing yourself half an hour for this series of morning 'rituals' really gets your mind and body set for the day. It makes you feels energized and buoys up your mood.

## AT DIFFERENT TIMES DURING THE DAY, WHILE TRAVELLING OR IN A WORK BREAK

Controlled breathing (pranayama) is the best way to recharge your mind and body. Slow, deep breathing is calming and yet invigorating, because it induces no feeling of lethargy or inertia. It helps you to connect to your inner self, almost meditatively, and through it you control your moods, your emotions and fatigue.

1 Blow your nose to clear your nasal passages. Sit straight, push your neck back a little to keep the cervical spine aligned.

2 Breathe in, gently bellowing out your abdomen. Hold your breath as you silently count to five.

3 Exhale slowly, again counting to five as you do so, while sucking your abdomen in.

Even in a workplace, where the air may not be fresh, this slow, gentle breathing increases your oxygen intake. It is easy but effective and only takes up 2–5 minutes a few times a day. After only a few weeks not only you but others will notice the difference, as the peace and calmness in your face cannot be hidden.

## Salutation to the sun

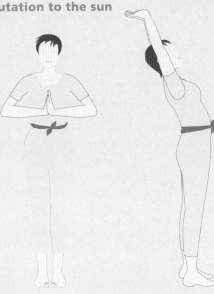

4 Breathe in and take your left leg back, resting the knee on the floor, with your toes curled under. Stretch your right knee forward while keeping the heel on the floor. Straighten your upper back and neck.

1 Stand with feet and palms together. Take a few slow, deep breaths and keep your shoulders down and neck straight.

2 Take a deep breath in, relax and expand your ribs outwards and forwards. Lift your arms and stretch back, pushing hips forwards but keeping legs straight.

3 Breathe out slowly and fold fowards, reaching down to place your palms on the floor. Lower your head towards your shins, relaxing your neck. If you can, straighten your legs.

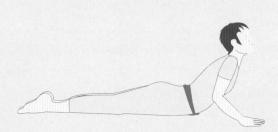

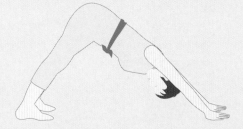

7 Breathe in and lower your hips to the floor. Point your toes and then stretch back. Press your shoulders down (you may need to bend your elbows), keep your upper back straight, push your chest forwards and look up.

8 Breathe out, curl your toes under again and lift your hips to form an upside-down 'V'. Stretch your heels down gently to touch the floor and relax your head down. Stretch out your arms and keep your spine straight.

5 Hold your breath and take your right foot back to join the left one. Support your weight on your hands and toes. Keep your spine in line with your head and look at the space in-between your hands.

6 Breathe out and lower your knees towards the floor by bending your arms. If your arms can't hold you, lower your knees to the floor first. Now lower your chest and forehead to the ground without dropping your hips.

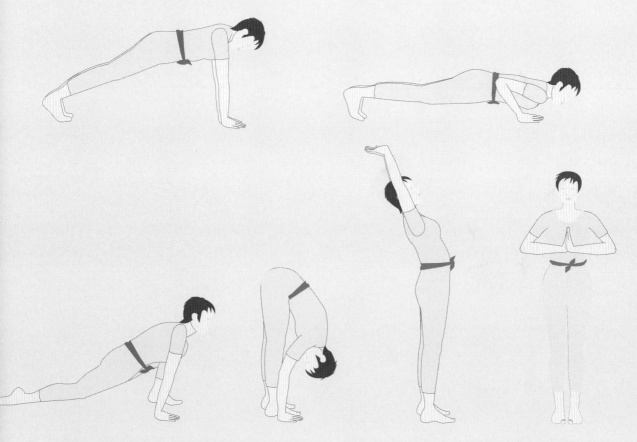

9 Breathe in and step your left foot forwards in-between your hands. Rest your right knee on the ground and straighten your neck, as in step 4.

10 Breathe out, bring your right foot forwards beside the left one, straighten your legs and fold forwards, as in step 3. Try to bend from the hips.

11 Breathe in, stretch your arms out in front of you and then left up and stretch back, as in step 2.

12 Breathe out and lower your arms into the prayer position. Stand straight and tall. You've completed 1 round; repeat and build gradually to 12 rounds.

## LUNCHTIME IN THE OFFICE

The second half of the day can be a strain. Most people struggle through it, often fuelled by coffee and snacks, and by the end of the day feel they need some alcohol 'to unwind'. Try relegating lunchtime chores to after work instead, and benefit from using the lunch period to regenerate your energy as follows.

If there is no quiet room in the office, put your head on your folded arms on the desk. Make sure you are not going to be disturbed by the phone or colleagues.

1 Consciously relax your neck and shoulder muscles. Breathe in and out as described in Exercise 3 (see Controlled Breathing, pages 73–4).

2 Focus on each part of your body in sequence, starting with your forehead and working down to your toes, then back to your forehead and out across your shoulders and down to your fingertips (see Relaxation, pages 73–4). Repeat both these cycles two or three times.

3 Let your eyelids relax, then your cheeks, your lips, your jaw and your throat. Say to yourself you feel calm and relaxed. Enjoy the state of relaxation and drift away to a space where there are no worries. You will wake up when you want to. Set your mind to a mental alarm of 5 or 10 minutes, depending on the time available to you.

4 Open your eyes and get up slowly. Wash your eyes, if you can.

This relaxation technique will refresh you for the afternoon.

## AT YOUR DESK

Using computers and sitting at a desk puts a lot of stress on the neck and shoulder area. Relieving this stress helps to reduce tension and enables a better flow of blood to the brain (see Massage, pages 66–9). Every three or four hours:

◆ Massage your neck and shoulder with your hands. Massage your jaw and eyes and gently press your ears as you did first thing in the morning. If you have been sitting in front of a computer, massage your arms from elbows up to the wrist.

◆ Grab your right shoulder with your left hand, keeping your shoulder parallel to your hips (i.e. don't twist). Pull your right shoulder forwards as you turn your head to look over it. Hold this position for a count of five. You may feel slight tension on the left side of the neck. Do the same with the left shoulder and right hand. Repeat three times.

◆ Drop your chin as far as you can towards your chest. Roll your head clockwise in a circular motion, making sure the circle is complete. Do this three times. Repeat the same anticlockwise.

## ON ARRIVING HOME

Walk around barefoot for a while. This relieves tension and eases your feet. If possible, take 15 minutes' time out. Taking this short time to unwind helps relieve physical fatigue, and gives you energy to enjoy your family and take on whatever domestic chores are waiting.

◆ Drink some water and lie on the bed or on the carpet with a cushion under your head. Close your eyes, relax; perhaps listen to a relaxing tape or CD.

◆ A few yoga stretches will ease the tension in your spine. Try the cobra (opposite) and boat and bridge (page 155). Three repeats of each will be enough.

## DURING THE EVENING

Spend three or four minutes on eye exercises:

- Keep your head still and look in sequence: straight up, obliquely up left, straight left, obliquely down left, straight obliquely down right, straight right and obliquely up right. Hold each gaze for three seconds. Repeat the full sequence three times.
- Rotate your eyeballs, following an imagined dot clockwise. Do this three times. Do the same anticlockwise three times.
- Rub your palms against each other till they get warm with friction. Apply your palms to your closed eyes to warm them.

## AFTER DINNER

The digestive system is very sluggish at night and so a little mild exercise helps. Walk about (indoors or out) for about 10 minutes to activate the intestines and aid digestion. Sleeping with a full stomach causes indigestion and insomnia and can contribute to weight problems.

## BEFORE GOING TO BED

- Lie on the floor and do 3–5 repetitions of the cobra, boat and semi-bridge poses (see above and page 155). These ease the muscles of the spine.
- Massage (or, better, get your partner to massage) your neck, shoulders, temples and scalp for two to three minutes in all. Once a week, extend this massage more fully (see Massage, pages 66–9).
- Facial massage will firm up the muscles and keep the skin toned. Gently massage your cheeks, jaw, forehead, eyebrows and eyes. Use some eye cream around your eyes so as not to drag the delicate skin.

## Cobra

1 Lie on your stomach with your feet together. Spread your arms out so that your hands are at ear level, in a straight line with your elbows, and rest your forehead on the ground.

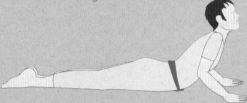

2 Breathe in and lift up your torso. Press your shoulders down and back. Look up, pushing your chest forwards. Come down slowly, breathing deeply. Repeat 5 times.

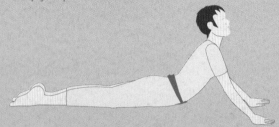

3 Over time, move into the full Cobra by straightening your arms, and work up to holding the post for 12 breaths. Breathe out and lower your forehead back to the floor.

## IF YOU WAKE UP IN THE NIGHT

- Go to the toilet, drink a glass of water.
- Massage your neck, shoulders, jaws, temples and ears.
- Do controlled retention breathing (as described on pages 73–4) and imagine that your legs and arms are relaxing, filling up with blood and feeling heavy.

This slow breathing and relaxation will soon send you back to sleep. Even if you don't sleep for very long, you'll feel very relaxed indeed.

# health, well-being and illness

It is my hope that by following the guidelines in the Lifestyle Programme that you will remain in good health and full of vitality. It is almost inevitable, however, that you will encounter health problems at some point in your life, and I hope that in the chapters in this section of the book you will find help and advice to overcome whatever may befall you. Prevention is undoubtedly the best medicine, but after that it is important to recognize as soon as possible any signs of impending ill-health, so that you can take prompt action – treatments are naturally more effective and need be less drastic if steps are taken at an early stage.

But this part of the book is not just about diseases and disorders. It covers the many things that affect a woman's body, from puberty to pregnancy, motherhood, the menopause and ageing. These are natural processes but they frequently have associated problems. Understanding what is going on within your body, and adapting to accommodate what is happening, is a vital part of enjoying rather than suffering the natural changes that are part of being a woman.

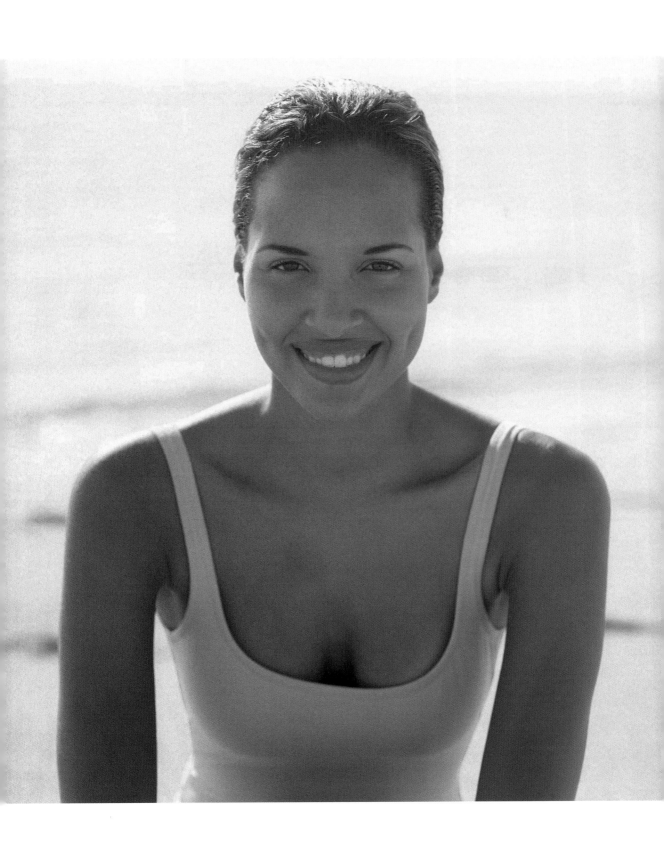

# chapter one

# reproductive health

From puberty into old age a woman's reproductive system affects her whole being. It influences her ability to conceive and her enjoyment of sex, her weight and the brittleness of her bones. The reverse is also true: a woman's general health has repercussions on her reproductive system. The reproduction process is controlled by the involuntary nervous system, which is linked to the body's energy system and healing power. Neglecting nutrition, exposing yourself to stress (which might be physical, emotional or environmental) or depriving yourself of rest will affect your well-being and have an adverse influence on your reproductive system.

# An anatomical guide
Take extra precautions to maintain your overall well-being, keep your mind and body in harmony and your reproductive system is likely to function well. Specific problems can often be traced back to general health.

Problems relating to the reproductive system have a deep impact on a woman's psyche. For example, if your period is delayed and you don't want to get pregnant the worry can affect your work, behaviour, energy and concentration; spotting between periods can generate worries about fibroids, hormonal imbalance, etc; and visiting a doctor about gynaecological problems can be a source of embarrassment.

## THE UTERUS AND CERVIX

With today's technology it's possible to grow an embryo outside the womb, or uterus, but under normal circumstances this is the organ where life is born. It provides nutrition and protection for a baby from shortly after conception until the moment of birth. The placenta, embedded in its walls, provides nutrients for the growing foetus and removes waste matter; the thick walls of the uterus and the fluid it contains (amniotic fluid) protect the unborn child, absorbing shocks and pressure; and the muscular uterine walls work to deliver the child when it is time to be born.

Although the uterus does not reach full development until puberty, it is there at birth and even begins to develop in the foetus from about 10 weeks. Because of its role to hold an unborn child, it is often imagined as a large organ, but unless you are pregnant it is only about 8cm long and 5cm wide. It is often described as pear-shaped, as it is roughly round but narrows into the cervical canal with an indented ring shape around the neck, or cervix, where it joins the vagina. (The vagina itself is covered in more detail in the chapter on Vaginal and Urinary Health.)

The uterus is sheathed in a thick membrane, an extension of the peritoneum, which covers and protects all the abdominal organs in one way or another. Strong

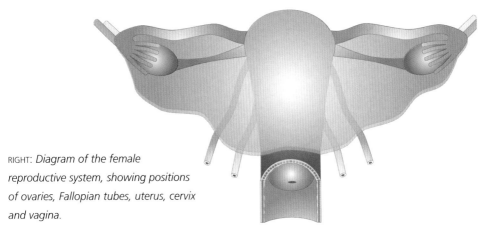

RIGHT: *Diagram of the female reproductive system, showing positions of ovaries, Fallopian tubes, uterus, cervix and vagina.*

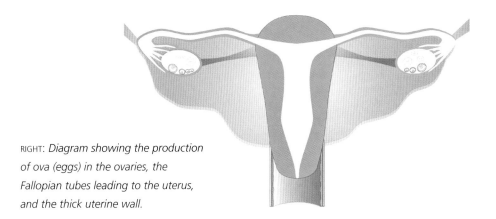

RIGHT: *Diagram showing the production of ova (eggs) in the ovaries, the Fallopian tubes leading to the uterus, and the thick uterine wall.*

ligaments hold the uterus in place, keeping it supported in pregnancy so that it remains freely suspended, despite the weight of the fluid and the growing baby.

In a woman of reproductive age who has not given birth, the uterine wall is about 2cm thick, consisting of an outer layer of involuntary muscles, the myometrium, and a thin inner layer, called the endometrium, which is jelly-like and full of blood vessels. One set of arteries reaches the endometrium from outside, passing through the myometrium, and another set encircles the endometrium. Its glands, blood vessels and other cells change under hormonal influences, each month growing and ripening, then shedding blood and tissue as menstruation.

## THE OVARIES AND FALLOPIAN TUBES

The two ovaries, each shaped like a miniature rugby ball, lie to left and right of the uterus. They are only about 3cm long during the reproductive years but each contains, amazingly, around 200,000 ovarian follicles. Each of these contains an egg (ovum). The ovaries also produce and are influenced by various reproductive hormones (see Ovarian and Uterine Cycles, below).

The ovaries are linked to the upper part of the uterus by a short tube, again one on each side, about 10cm long. These are the Fallopian tubes, also known as oviducts, because it is through these that an egg travels

to the uterus upon ovulation each month. The ends of the tubes are fringed, to 'catch' the egg as it is released by the ovary, and it is in a Fallopian tube that, if successfully penetrated by sperm, an egg is fertilized. The tubes have a frond-like lining, which helps the egg move along the tube to the uterus.

## HEALTH CHECKS

The uterus is the site of common cancers (cervical and myometrial) and regular checks are recommended to all women who are or have been sexually active. These may be annually or every three years. A manual gynaecological examination will feel for hard or unusual tissue or incipient tumours in the uterus, and a cervical smear (called a Pap smear) will be taken to look for any abnormal cell development on the cervix. Being told that abnormal cells have been found can be frightening, but they do not mean that you have cancer. They will simply indicate that further checks should be made (which may involve nothing more than smears at more frequent intervals) and it is quite usual for subsequent tests to be negative. If any pre-cancerous cells are confirmed, the disease will have been caught at a very early stage if you have been regularly checked in the past.

• *See also Giving Yourself an MOT (pages 37–47).*

# Menstruation Understanding the amazing synchronization of different parts of your system helps to explain what might be happening when things go wrong.

## Ovarian and uterine cycles

Although monthly periods are often an inconvenience and bring with them discomfort and mood swings, they are an indication that the reproductive cycle is working. A complex but minutely orchestrated combination of hormonal impulses creates the reproductive cycles that ensure that everything happens as it should.

The hypothalamus secretes GnRH (gonadotrophin releasing hormone) at certain intervals and volumes (known as frequency and amplitude). This rhythm of GnRH secretion is called the pulse.

When the GnRH pulse reaches 16–24 per day (one pulse every 60–90 minutes), the pituitary secretes FSH (follicle stimulating hormone), which signals the ovarian follicle to develop and secrete oestrogen. The rising level of oestrogen in the blood triggers the hypothalamus to secrete more GnRH and the pulse rises further. At about 36 per day, the pituitary secretes another hormone, LH (luteinizing hormone), and together FSH and LH trigger the development of an egg follicle. (Incidentally, usually only one ovary at a time responds, even though the hormones target them both.)

When the quickening pulse arrives every 30 minutes, the egg follicle, which has now reached a diameter of about 15mm, bulges out of the ovary like a balloon and bursts, releasing the egg, which is drawn towards the funnel of the Fallopian tube. Here it may be fertilized.

## ONE MESSENGER, MANY MESSAGES

Our body's reaction to a hormonal impulse is quite different from a nervous one. Our nerves stimulate a single reaction – we sense the heat of a flame, we pull our hand away – our knee is tapped in a particular place, the lower leg swings up. A hormonal stimulus acts simultaneously on relevant parts of our body. If we see a mugger coming for us, the hormone adrenalin causes our heart to race, our lungs to breathe faster, our muscles to tense ready for running, our liver to release glucose for instant energy, our pancreas to secrete cortisol and adrenalin and our cells to release energy molecules – one messenger, many messages.

The source of the message is in the brain, specifically the hypothalamus. The hypothalamus sends some messages directly through the nervous system but triggers others by releasing messenger hormones. It sends these out either directly or instructs the pituitary, which lies just below it, to do so. (The adrenalin that allows us to escape the mugger is triggered by the pituitary's instruction to the adrenal glands.)

In the case of the reproductive cycles, the ovarian hormones work in concert to bring about the most phenomenal changes, triggering egg development, growth of uterine cells, endometrial glands and blood vessels in the uterus and then, in the case of an unfertilized egg, the disintegration of the endometrium.

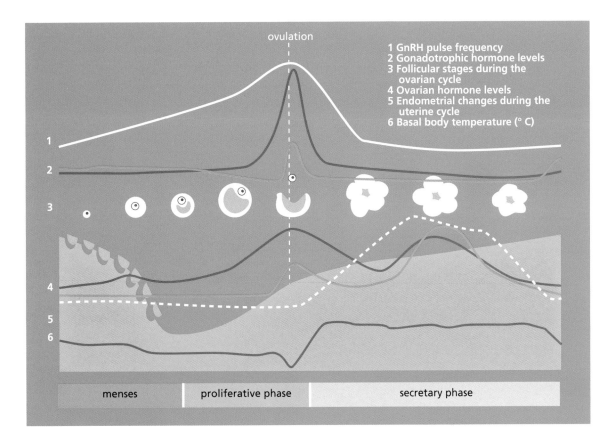

ovulation

1 GnRH pulse frequency
2 Gonadotrophic hormone levels
3 Follicular stages during the
  ovarian cycle
4 Ovarian hormone levels
5 Endometrial changes during the
  uterine cycle
6 Basal body temperature (° C)

1
2
3
4
5
6

menses | proliferative phase | secretary phase

Occasionally, more than one follicle ripens and releases an egg. Should both (or, more rarely, three or more) eggs be fertilized, this will be the beginning of fraternal (non-identical) twins or triplets.

The developed follicle, which had up to now been 'squashing' all other ovarian tissue to stop any other follicles developing, shrinks back on bursting and gradually forms a hard mass called the 'corpus luteum', or luteal body.

In the meantime, the high level of LH also triggers secretion of another ovarian hormone, progesterone. Under the influence of oestrogen, the endometrium has been building up since the last menstrual period, but this increase in progesterone stimulates more rapid development, in preparation for a fertilized egg. This phase of rapid growth of the endometrium lasts for approximately 14 days, at which point the endometrium is fully developed.

If the released egg has been fertilized, the corpus luteum (i.e. the remnant of the ovarian follicle the egg came from) continues to secrete progesterone; if not, secretion is switched off. When the endometrium stops getting any hormonal instructions and support from the ovary its spiral arteries constrict. Just as, when you cut a branch off a tree, the leaves on it wither away, the endometrial cells begin to die off in patches. The blood vessels in the spiral arteries begin to rupture. This, coupled with necrotized tissue, causes the entire endometrium to collapse. This is the onset of menstruation.

The repair work starts as soon as the bleeding ends, as new cells begin to grow and another cycle begins.

## PULSE DIAGNOSIS

Until the mid-1930s most physicians were taught and used pulse diagnosis. Today it is a forgotten art. I have been using pulse diagnosis for over twenty years and, having mastered the art to some degree, am teaching doctors to use it in their practices. They have been astonished to observe how the nature of the pulse changes in women who are pregnant or menstruating or ovulating, going through premenstrual tension or are anaemic.

If the pulse indicates the stage of the menstrual cycle and uterine function, the body must be going through other changes too: the reproductive cycle is not isolated. The respiratory, digestive, hormonal, renal, circulatory, metabolic and emotional functions are deeply involved, and any abnormality is bound to be reflected in the function of the entire body and mind. Some symptoms which can only be assessed subjectively, such as fatigue, lack of concentration, emotional changes, memory loss or sleep disturbances, are often brushed off as 'mental' conditions by physicians, yet they form part and parcel of the reproductive cycle.

# That time of the month

Even though menstruation is a normal physiological occurrence, it puts the body's energy reserve and healing power under some strain. Too often women concentrate on the practicalities such as hygiene and totally ignore the implication it has on their wider health.

It is a misconception that you lose a lot of blood during normal menstruation: only about 40–50ml of blood is lost, and endometrial cells (i.e. from the lining of the uterus) constitute the rest. The sloughing of endometrial tissue is gradual, which is why menstruation usually lasts three to five days, but can be up to a week.

Menstrual blood should be dark red in colour, but without pieces of dark brown clots. It has a strong odour because, unlike fresh blood, it is not flowing directly from veins or arteries. It also contains dead tissue from the endometrium that has begun to 'necrotize' or die back a few days before.

Symptoms accompanying menstruation can be minimal or profound: two or three days bedridden with migraine, or period pains more severe than labour pains. Conventional medicine treats these debilitating conditions symptomatically, regarding them as hormonal problems even after blood tests reveal normal hormone levels; and in most cases, when progesterone is administered, there is no improvement. It is obvious that we have to look for the answers elsewhere.

## COSSET YOURSELF

Advertisements for tampons and sanitary pads stress the ability to be 'carefree' during periods, but in fact these days are exactly when you do need to care for yourself. Although the loss of blood is not great, the days around the start of a period may bring on discomfort or pain, difficult mood swings and you may feel generally drained – not without reason is a common expression for the menstrual period 'the curse'. In India, women were traditionally exempt from praying, going to temples, cooking, carrying babies, carrying water pitchers, meeting too many people and so on for the first three days of their periods. (The use of cosmetics, massage, swimming, shouting, sitting in strong wind, listening to loud music, arguing, and standing for long hours were also not recommended, and sexual contact or even arousal was not permitted.)

In modern times, such precautions are hard to take. There is no provision in the employment law to take time off during these critical days, and generally women want to be discreet about their periods.

## Things that help

A light, easily digestible diet, to avoid straining your body and sapping energy. Home-made chicken soup, fish, chicken, eggs, soaked almonds, carrots and apple juice, pomegranate, raw salad, potatoes, rice, pasta and green vegetables are all good.

- **Warm showers or a bath** once or twice a day if possible. Personal hygiene at this time is very important.

- **A good fluid intake**: 2 litres of water a day. Teas such as fennel, mint or basil can help you relax, especially if they are made from fresh leaves. (Boil herb leaves for 2–3 minutes, add ordinary tea leaves if wished, strain and add honey to taste.)

- **Relaxation.** Tension, both physical and mental, exacerbates symptoms and stress is likely to be magnified by the hormonal changes your body is undergoing, even if you don't actually suffer from PMS (see page 100). So stretch out and rest whenever you can, listen to quiet music and do anything that will keep you feeling calm. Malty drinks are relaxing, and some people believe that even wearing certain colours, such as white, lilac, pink and turquoise, can lift your mood.

- **Controlled breathing** (see box).

If your periods naturally tend to be heavy, you may need to take a day or two off as part of sick leave or unpaid leave. Consult your GP if this becomes a long-term problem. Anything strenuous (long hours at a computer, carrying, lifting and standing for a long time) becomes a great strain and is not advisable.

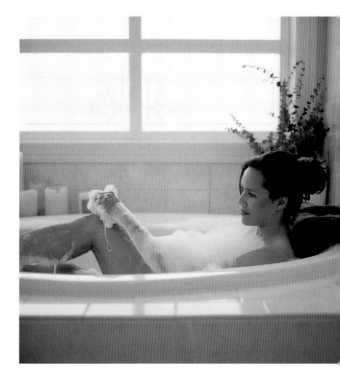

## Breathing exercise

Spending a minute or two on this every couple of hours or so helps to calm the mind and oxygenates the blood better.
- Loosen your clothing and lie comfortably on your back.
- Breathe in slowly and deeply over three seconds, bellowing out your abdomen as you do so (this may be the opposite of what you usually do as you inhale).
- Hold your breath for a further three seconds and then slowly breathe out over six seconds, sucking in your abdomen as you do so.
- Repeat 10 times.

*For more on controlled breathing, see the Lifestyle Programme.*

## Things that don't help

- **Food that is heavy to digest:** fried food, sausages, bacon, butter, curries, chillies, red meat, offal

- Citrus fruit

- Ice cream, chilled drinks, ice cubes

- Smoking

- Coffee

- Alcohol

- Tight-fitting clothes

- **Travelling,** general stress at work and home, irregular hours etc.

## PERIOD PAINS

This is the most uncomfortable symptom of periods. Sometimes the pain is so severe that women pass out, and as many as 20 per cent of girls take time off school because of period pains (although this is a difficult statistic to ascertain). Pains usually last for one or two days before and during the period and vary both in intensity and type. Some women experience a dull, nagging ache in the abdomen and lower back; others have sharp cramping and tenderness across the lower abdomen; for others the pain is 'colicky', coming and going in waves. These different types of pain have different causes.

Misaligned uterus: The uterus is held in suspension by ligaments. Sometimes, either due to nutrition or genetic predisposition, these ligaments are not strong enough and the uterus is tilted too far either forwards or backwards. This results in the formation of a kink in or near the neck of the uterus. At the beginning of a

# SEX

This is a tricky time for women. The neck of the uterus is dilated to facilitate the menstrual flow, which increases the chance of infection reaching the uterus. Sexual contact or even excitement or arousal also puts a lot of strain on a woman's body.

For couples who are used to regular lovemaking, abstaining for a week may create tension. The matter gets worse if you have PMS for a week, when you may not wish to be touched, and then you have another week of abstinence. Exciting yourself for your partner's sake is not a good idea, and if you have the space it may be easier to sleep in a separate room for these days. Talk this through together to avoid misunderstandings (men can often take personally a refusal or lack of interest in sex).

Your period is the end of one cycle but also the beginning of the next. As soon as the endometrium has shed its old lining it begins to rebuild a new one, to be prepared if a fertilized egg should arrive. This rebuilding calls for a blood supply and for you to supply good-quality raw materials (through nutrients).

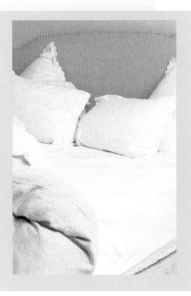

period, the blood cannot pass easily past this kink, so the uterus begins to contract, as if in labour, to force the menstrual flow on its way. This is when intense waves of pain start. This type of period pain is debilitating and even strong painkillers do not help, but it stops suddenly as soon as the blood has been expelled beyond the kink.

Such period pains most commonly start in late adolescence. The contraceptive pill is frequently prescribed to control the pains but it won't help if the problem is structural. Childbirth often realigns the uterus, which is why, when periods start again, they often come without pain.

Sore abdominal tendons: Another source of pain is the tendons that attach the lower ends of the abdominal muscles to the pubic bone. These tendons can get inflamed and sore from excessive exercise of certain sorts (sit-ups, weights, riding a bicycle, kickboxing, step machine) or from increased pressure on them from weight gain or an abdomen bloated from pelvic congestion just before a period. The result is severe lower abdominal pain until the period starts.

## Treatments

Pain from whatever source will be exacerbated by strain and tension. Follow the general advice for during periods (see Cosseting Yourself, page 90–1). Stick to food that is easy to digest and in particular steer clear of everything on the 'Things that don't help' list. High stomach acids may affect the collagen in tendons and ligaments, so if your lower abdomen is tender avoid citrus fruit.

### Easing cramps:

◆ When the cramps start, massage the area just above the pubic bone, using peppermint balm (which is especially soothing), tiger balm or simply olive or sesame oil. Massage gently and then with a slight pressure. This relieves the soreness in the tendons in this area, and results can be dramatic.

## UNEXPECTED PAINS

If you suddenly experience period pains, when you have not had them in the past, they may be a symptom of an infection of the uterus lining, or irritation caused by, for example, an intra-uterine device (contraceptive coil). This should be checked out straight away by your GP or clinic.

◆ Drink malty drinks and calming herbal tea with honey – try chamomile or peppermint. Avoid very cold drinks.

### A pain-relieving poultice:

◆ Heat 1 cup of salt in a pan for five minutes or so. Pour the salt in the centre of a tea towel or square of cloth. Tie it up to make a poultice (wrap in another layer if the contents are too hot). Dab this hot poultice on the lower part of your abdomen, particularly just above the pubic bone. Do this for five minutes or so three times a day. To make the poultice even more potent, add 1 teaspoon of mustard seeds or thyme, and heat together with the salt.

### Supplements:

Homeopathic remedies can be helpful:

◆ pulsatilla 30: suck two tablets three times a day. Begin two days before the expected start of your period and continue for the first day or two of your period. Do this for three or four cycles to get results.
◆ belladonna 30: suck two tablets every two hours while the cramps continue.

## EXCESSIVE BLEEDING (MENORRHAGIA)

Some women have naturally light periods, while others regularly lose much more blood but still fall within the range of what is considered normal. Very heavy or prolonged periods (over more than seven days), which may be characterized by 'gushing' and clots, indicate the uterus is continuing to bleed after it has done its normal shedding of the blood-engorged endometrium. This extra blood loss can be debilitating, causing anaemia, headaches, dizziness, fatigue and fainting.

The cause may be a chronic, and perhaps undetected condition such as fibroids or endometriosis (see pages 110–11 and 104–6), or it may be brought on by the fitting of an IUD (contraceptive coil). An unusually excessive period may be a symptom of a tumour, or a prolapsed uterus, or even a miscarriage, and should always be investigated.

### Treatments

If no specific cause has been diagnosed, the bleeding over and above the usual menstrual blood has to be stopped. Do not work or carry anything heavy. Bed-rest helps and you should move only when absolutely necessary. Ice packs on the lower abdomen will help contract the uterus and staunch the flow.

Compensate for the loss of blood with a highly nutritious diet to help the blood regenerate as soon as possible.

◆ Eat plenty of protein, such as meat and poultry. Vegetarians should eat eggs; vegans should get as much protein as possible from soaked almonds, other high-protein nuts such as cashews and peanuts (choose unsalted ones), soya products and ghee.

◆ Have two cups a day of home-made chicken stock (see page 65).

◆ Other good sources of blood-synthesizing elements are organic calf or chicken liver, and pomegranate.

◆ Juiced carrot and red apple with a little root ginger helps to tone up the body and prevent low blood pressure and consequent fatigue.

*Supplements:*

◆ supari pak, an ayurvedic supplement made from betel nuts, helps the uterine wall to contract gently. This squeezes the numerous blood vessels that penetrate the muscular uterine wall, allowing the blood to clot.

◆ lachesis 30 and sepia 30. Take alternately every two hours or as recommended by a homeopath. (Illustrating the homeopathic principle of treating like with like, lachesis is a snake venom that causes haemorrhaging but in minute homeopathic doses it has the opposite effect.)

◆ Indian unani remedies, such as bandish khoon, are also very effective if you can take them under appropriate medical supervision.

## SCANTY PERIODS (OLIGOMENORRHEA)

This is a pattern of periods when they are over 35 days apart and less than three days in duration. If you think it unlikely you have reached the menopause (although this can be premature), such light periods may be an indication of poor nutrition, lack of ovulation or polycystic ovaries.

### Treatments

Follow the dietary advice in the Lifestyle Programme, and:

◆ ensure you are getting plenty of protein. Vegans, in particular, or teenage girls who are eating too little in an effort to lose weight, can be missing out on vital nutrients.

◆ include in your diet: pomegranate, rhubarb, yam, avocado.

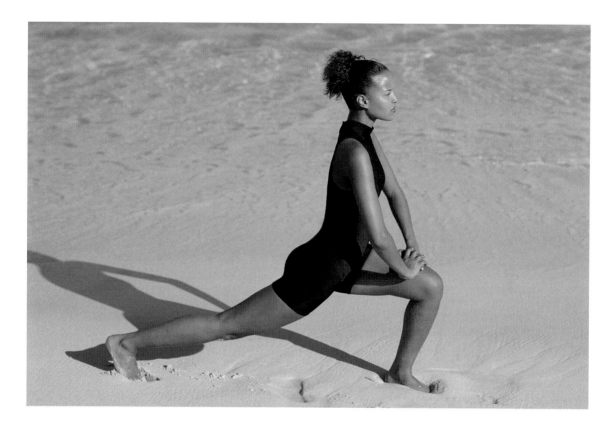

◆ check your diet is not low in fat-soluble vitamins. These help with hormonal regulation, particularly vitamin E in its natural form (rich sources are wheatgerm, vegetable oils, nuts and seeds).

◆ Fresh aloe vera can be beneficial (see amenorrhoea, below).

Stress can have an adverse effect on your periods, and for this I advise:

◆ neck and shoulder massage: at least two 10-minute sessions a week at home, or professionally three times a month

◆ acupuncture

◆ therapeutic yoga for stress management and to improve the functioning of the pituitary.

Sometimes the pill can be helpful in regulating periods.

*Supplements:*

◆ shatavari, dong quai and agnus castus, together with Mexican yam. These are oestrogen and progesterone mimics. What I prescribe is to take shatavari (1 tablet twice a day), dong quai (1 tablet a day) and agnus castus (10 drops) for 15 days after the end of your period. Then take a capsule of Mexican yam until your next period starts. This way you will take no supplements during the periods.

◆ phyto-oestrogens. There are several available: consult an integrated medical physician or qualified herbalist.

◆ several homeopathic remedies are beneficial: consult a qualified homeopath.

## LACK OF PERIODS (AMENORRHOEA)

Your periods naturally stop when you become pregnant or reach the menopause, but other factors can cause them to dry up in a woman whose menstruation has previously been normal. When this absence of periods extends to six months or more, it is termed secondary amenorrhoea. (Primary amenorrhoea indicates that menstruation has never started: see box opposite.)

Almost all women can ovulate by stimulation with drugs but not all can conceive, especially without proper periods, so a lack of periods is a major worry for those who want to have children.

Nutritional deficiencies, severe weight loss, excessive exercise and sudden trauma can all cause periods to cease, especially when they affect the balance of one or more reproductive hormones. Disorders such as anaemia and Crohn's disease (causing diarrhoea and nutritional imbalance) can also result in cessation of periods.

## ANOREXIA NERVOSA

Although the root of this condition is psychological, a common effect is amenorrhoea, brought on by chronic lack of nutrition, often coupled with extended bouts of demanding physical exercise (see the chapter on Psychological Health).

### Diet and exercise

◆ Crash diets, anorexia or being markedly underweight from illness or stress can result in the loss of periods. Very restrictive diets, especially if avoiding animal protein or any sort of fats, can cause a deficiency of the fat-soluble vitamins, A, D, E and K. Vitamin E is very important for women, and if the body is short of essential fats (particularly cholesterol) the synthesis of oestrogen is affected.

◆ Lack of iron, resulting in anaemia and very low blood pressure, makes the body sluggish and it will attempt to protect itself from any blood loss. Anaemic conditions also affect the function of the pituitary gland, which triggers certain hormonal secretions.

◆ Many high-level sportswomen, exercise instructors, ballerinas, and women involved in heavy physical work find their periods stop at times of intense training because, as a result of building up muscle bulk, the adrenal glands secrete steroids that are similar to male hormones in nature.

### Hormonal imbalance

◆ Physical trauma – head injury, whiplash, even excessive dental work or a complication that dates back to birth (forceps, ventouse delivery, etc.) – can reduce the blood flow through the vertebral arteries in the neck. This can impair the performance of the pituitary–hypothalamic area of the brain, vital to hormone secretion.

◆ Severe stress – bereavement, illness, divorce, major financial difficulties – can cause the adrenal glands to be over-stimulated and the pituitary to be exhausted. Stress hormones (adrenalin/noradrenalin) are like androgens (male hormones) in nature and so can interfere with normal female cycles.

◆ A poorly functioning thyroid, a pituitary tumour or certain drugs such as dopamine antagonists can cause an increase in prolactin levels. Prolactin is the

# PRIMARY AMENORRHOEA

About 98 per cent of girls have begun their normal menstrual cycle by the age of 16. If other signs of puberty (pubic hair, breast development, etc.) are normal but there are no periods, this is called primary amenorrhoea. Causes include:

- a genetic abnormality in the reproductive organs, such as an underdeveloped uterus or vagina; occasionally the hymen is totally closed, allowing no menstrual flow
- an atrophied endometrium (womb lining – see page 102)

- anomalies in the pituitary–hypothalamic area, the brain's hormone-regulating zone. If the pituitary does not secrete the hormones that stimulate the ovaries, these in turn won't secrete oestrogen, the main facilitator of periods. Anomalies might include defective blood vessels in the hypothalamus or a pituitary tumour
- polycystic ovaries (see page 107).

See also Premature and Delayed Puberty (page 102).

hormone that triggers breast-milk production, and so overrides the usual hormonal signals that control ovulation and menstruation.

- Some scientists believe that leptin, the hormone that controls weight gain, plays an important role in regulating menstruation. They argue that anorexics do not menstruate because leptin production is low; when they gain weight their periods return. My personal view is that this is primarily a matter of nutritional imbalance.

## Disease

- Polycystic ovary syndrome (PCOS) is often character-ized by menstrual irregularities (see page 107–8).
- The liver metabolizes oestrogens and is instrumental in the conversion of excess androgens (male hormones) to oesterone (a relative of oestrogen). Liver diseases such as hepatitis and cirrhosis can interfere with these processes, resulting in too many male hormones in the body.
- Disorders that affect the digestion and absorption of nutrients, such as anaemia, ulcerative colitis and Crohn's disease, and result in dramatic weight loss, are often accompanied by loss of periods.

## Treatments

Whatever the root cause, amenorrhoea is usually symptomatic of a nutritional or hormonal imbalance, often both interlinked. The sooner you start treatment, the better the results are. Do not wait for six months for your doctor to confirm the diagnosis of amenorrhoea. If you do not have periods for two months (and are not pregnant or menopausal), do something about it. This integrated treatment plan of diet, massage, relaxation and supplements has helped many women with secondary amenorrhoea and some with primary amenorrhoea.

*Nutrition:*

- A high-protein diet is essential: eat eggs, fish, poultry and lean meat. Vegetable proteins are not so effective in this treatment plan: to kick-start periods you need more than cottage cheese, soya products such as tofu, and nuts and lentils.
- Take folic acid and iron as well as multivitamins and minerals as general supplements.
- Pomegranates, apples, cherries, yam, rhubarb, avocado and nuts (especially almonds, pistachios, Brazil nuts and hazelnuts) all provide vitamins and minerals helpful to restoring menstruation.

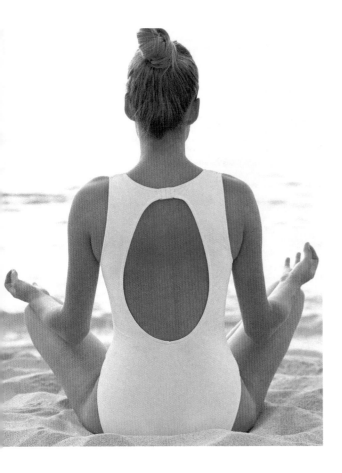

*Supplements:*

◆ zinc: one 15mg tablet every other day for two months.

◆ shatavari (1 tablet twice daily), dong quai (1 tablet daily) and agnus castus (10–15 drops daily) for the first half of the calendar month, then Mexican yam (1 capsule twice daily) and shatavari (1 tablet daily) for the second half of the calendar month. This alternating pattern of oestrogen-mimics in the first half of the month and then progesterone-mimics in the second half can help trigger the return of periods.

◆ aloe vera: one capsule twice daily, or one teaspoonful of fresh gel or pulp. Do not take the latter if you are pregnant, or think you may be.

*Other aids:*

◆ Acupuncture and homeopathy are useful in treating secondary amenorrhoea.

## VERY SHORT CYCLES (POLYMENORRHOEA)

Periods that occur more frequently than about every twenty-five days are usually due to lack of ovulation – if ovulation does not occur, then there is no need for the endometrium to grow, so it just breaks down.

### Treatments

Regular neck and shoulder massage helps to improve the functions of the pituitary gland (see pages 66–9 for details of why this works, and techniques). Homeopathy and acupuncture are also very useful.

*Supplements:*

◆ shatavari contains natural phyto-oestrogens, which help with menstrual functions.

◆ aloe vera capsules taken twice daily is a useful remedy.

◆ dong quai is a useful Chinese remedy.

*Massage:*

◆ The massage section of the Lifestyle Programme explains how neck and shoulder massage are effective in enhancing the function of the hypothalamus and pituitary. Have this treatment every other day if you have a willing partner, or else once a week by a trained massage therapist.

*Relaxation:*

◆ Try to minimize your stress levels. Resolving outside stresses may take a long time, but relaxation techniques will help you cope better with them. Yoga, meditation, and simply setting aside time for yourself to be quiet and perhaps listen to specially recorded tapes or CDs are all useful.

## IRREGULAR PERIODS (MENOMETRORRHAGIA)

Sometimes, bleeding occurs at irregular intervals and the duration and amount can also vary: periods appear to be all over the place and their very cyclical nature ceases to exist. Because this indicates bleeding from a cause in addition to menstruation, you must get this investigated to rule out anything such as a tumour or an undiagnosed pregnancy that has gone wrong.

When everything seems normal, doctors usually prescribe contraceptive pills to regulate the cycle. The hormones in the pill take over and the body's own hormones become ineffective. Unpredictable periods cause a lot of stress as their onset can be sudden and sometimes embarrassing, so the artificial cycle helps to bring in some law and order and provides relief.

### Treatments

When no cause has been found, I recommend the following:

- neck and shoulder massage (see pages 66–7) – very important.
- plenty of protein, such as meat and poultry. Vegetarians should eat eggs; vegans should get as much protein as possible from soaked almonds and other high-protein nuts (cashews and peanuts are the highest), soya products, ghee, etc.
- supari pak, as soon as bleeding starts or take it for three cycles continuously. This ayurvedic medicine helps stop uterine bleeding by encouraging the uterine wall to contract gently. This squeezes the numerous blood vessels that penetrate the muscular uterine wall, allowing the blood to clot.
- vigorous gym exercises (aerobics, light weights) and swimming. The natural steroids that intense exercise releases help to slow down bleeding (the same mechanism that causes scanty or missing periods in sportswomen in heavy training).

## BLEEDING BETWEEN PERIODS (METRORRHAGIA)

A one-off occasion of bleeding between periods is not a cause for concern, but if it repeats itself during the next cycle, you need to get it investigated. Consult a gynaecologist to identify the cause and get treatment. This type of bleeding is not connected to menstruation, and polyps, endometriosis (see pages 104–6), cancers, and erosion of the cervix are all possible causes. Hormone replacement therapy (HRT) can also lead to this type of bleeding at times.

### Treatments

If no cause has been found after investigation and the bleeding continues regularly, then follow the advice for excessive bleeding (menorrhagia) on page 94.

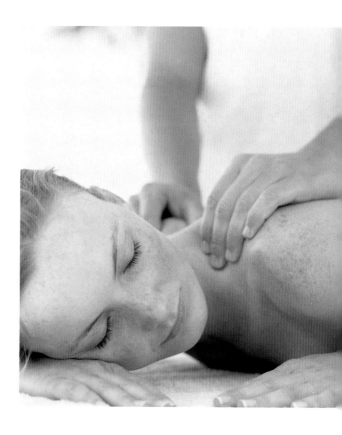

# Premenstrual syndrome (PMS) This is a controversial cluster of symptoms which strike in the second half of the menstrual cycle.

Up to 75 per cent of women experience these symptoms, which are particularly prevalent in women in their late twenties and early thirties.

## Symptoms

PMS varies greatly. For some women its symptoms are primarily physical: discomfort and bloating, while for others it means an uncharacteristic irritability and short temper, or an overpowering lethargy and trouble with concentrating or making decisions. It can manifest itself in uncontrollable mood swings or emotional hypersensitivity. Women who are calm, intelligent and rational suddenly become just the opposite.

These dramatic symptoms disappear again as soon as the period starts. It is this yo-yo or Jekyll and Hyde pattern that has fascinated me. Many men I have interviewed say this is the worst aspect of their partner: however beautiful, however kind she is, the irrational and unpredictable behaviour in the days leading up to her period makes it difficult for family and friends to cope. Severe PMS can endanger or break relationships; it can damage your self-confidence ('How could I have done/said that?') and your reputation at work. In the UK (but seldom in the USA), court cases for minor offences or antisocial behaviour have been successfully defended on the basis of PMS being a temporary disturbance to the state of mind.

It is interesting to note that PMS and chronic fatigue syndrome have many identical symptoms, except that the former is a short-term condition and irritability is a dominant symptom while CFS is characterized by extreme fatigue and depression (see pages 272–4).

## THE CURSE OF PMS

As many as 150 symptoms have been recorded, the majority of which are in the realm of psychological or behavioural patterns. Typical and common ones include:

- mood swings
- irritability
- water retention or bloating
- dizziness
- headaches
- breast tenderness
- pelvic pain
- chronic fatigue
- sleep disturbances
- clumsiness
- food cravings
- memory loss
- lack of concentration
- tearfulness
- poor libido

## Causes

The personality-altering nature of PMS might be likened to the effect that alcohol or recreational drugs have on loosening inhibitions, or that steroids have on heightening aggression, but with the source coming from within. Many theories involving hormonal imbalances, hypoglycaemia, psychogenic factors and other causes have been proposed to explain PMS and none fits the bill totally. The fact that PMS disappears when ovaries are surgically removed (because of cysts or cancer, for instance) or drugs suppress their function tends to confirm the hypothesis supported by most scientists that ovarian functions are the root cause.

My personal view is that damage control and preventive measures can go a long way towards mitigating the effects of PMS. The one thing about the condition is that it is usually predictable in its timing. You come to recognize the signs, you (and your family) know how you are likely to react and many women have learnt that there are particular triggers that make things worse. There are several steps you can take to dampen the symptoms or even make them disappear.

### Neck and shoulder massage

Of all of the treatments that I recommend, this is the most beneficial. I believe that before periods, the blood depot shifts to the pelvic region (a similar phenomenon occurs after a heavy meal, when the abdomens draw in extra blood to aid the digestive process). This is called pelvic congestion. This shift reduces the brain's supply of blood, and therefore the oxygen and glucose it needs. This supply is further restricted when the neck muscles are tight (due to general stress, insomnia) or the neck vertebrae misaligned. The reactions that this deprivation causes range across the entire gamut of PMS symptoms, from headaches, sugar cravings and panic attacks to mood swings and fatigue. Disturbance in the balance of the diuretic hormone governed by the hypothalamus accounts for the water retention and bloating.

For the massage technique, see Lifestyle Programme. Ask your partner to do this for you once a day for 10–15 minutes if the PMS is severe, or see someone professionally at least once during that period.

### Diet

I usually recommend a fairly restricted diet during the time that you get PMS. Be as easy on your digestive system as possible: the less strain on the digestion, the better your body in general feels. Avoid foods that may cause

- indigestion: fried food, citrus fruit
- water retention: salt
- bloating: mushrooms, cheese, yeast products
- excitement of the nervous system: ginger, excess salt
- fatigue: yeast products
- tension or irritability: coffee, alcohol
- cravings: sugary food.

Also avoid canned and preserved food, which are often high in salt and sugar and commonly contain preservatives, which may affect mood or have unknown effects. The main dietary guidelines in the Lifestyle Programme give more detailed explanations of the effects certain foods have on your body and mind.

Drink chamomile and other calming herbal teas.

Do regular therapeutic yoga (see Lifestyle Programme).
Listen to a relaxation tape or CD before you go to bed.

### Supplements:

- Take a B-complex vitamin daily (the B group are anti-stress vitamins).
- Gokhru tea helps with water retention.

# Health problems relating to the reproductive system
Maintaining the health of the reproductive system is of enormous importance, but problems can still occur, from endometriosis to fibroids to infertility.

## Premature and delayed puberty

Puberty is divided into three phases: first the breasts begin to develop (thelarche), then pubic and armpit hair begin to grow (pubarche) and the third stage is when menstruation begins (menarche). From the age of seven, there is a slow increase in sex hormones in the body, and puberty occurs between 8 and 13 in girls. Both boys and girls are reaching puberty earlier nowadays; it is estimated that the age is decreasing by between one and three months every decade.

Unless the body is put under strain in some way – perhaps by nutritional deficiencies or excessive exercise – the body will develop naturally and although girls will extensively compare notes and may fret about early or slow development, there is seldom anything to worry about.

However, puberty delayed beyond the age of 17 is a concern. The hormones relating to breast development, menstruation and so on are controlled by the pituitary–hypothalamic area of the brain, and the pituitary is also responsible for growth hormones. An absence of pubertal development and dwarfism often go together, indicating a malfunction of the pituitary–hypothalamic area. When periods do begin, the growth in height is restored also.

The hormone that controls weight gain, leptin, may also play a role in the development of puberty. Some scientists reason that anorexics do not menstruate because they lose weight and so leptin production is low (and their periods start again once they start eating regularly), and therefore an over-production of leptin, as happens in obesity, may contribute to early puberty.

Unusual pituitary function can also bring about another abnormality during puberty: adrenarche. Normally, the female hormone oestrogen dominates, but in this condition there is an over-secretion of adrenal male hormones (androgens). What causes this abnormality is unknown. I once treated a very young girl who had signs of adrenarche at the age of five, developing pubic hair, excess body hair and a strong body odour characteristic of the problem. Neck and back massage improved blood supply to the brain. When she began to grow I knew this was a sign that the pituitary was functioning better and would regulate the adrenal glands. Sure enough, the adrenarche was arrested.

### Treatments

Normal medical treatment involves the use of growth hormones and the pill, but these may not be right at that delicate age.

I use supplements to encourage correct hormonal stimulation: shatavari, dong quai and agnus cactus for the first 15 days of the calendar month and then a switch to Mexican yam for the last 15 days.

## Growing up too soon

At the age of five, Meena had lemon-sized breasts, pubic hair and had some spotting of blood. She developed a complex and would not go to school. Her parents were absolutely devastated. She was put on drugs to block the hormones.

I advised the parents to change her diet to include more protein, ginger, garlic and avocado, and taught them the neck and shoulder massage techniques that improve blood flow to the hormone-controlling areas of the brain (see pages 66–9). I also supplemented her diet with multivitamin and mineral tablets for general health and encouraged the family to go on walks every day (Meena was too embarrassed by her breasts to go swimming).

Within three months, her periods had stopped and her breasts had stopped growing. The pubic hair remained the same, but was scanty. I have treated about six other children in the same way, and I am confident that this treatment worked because of self-regulation of the pituitary–hypothalamic functions.

# Endometriosis

This is a condition in which the inner lining of the womb (endometrium) begins to appear in patches beyond the womb. As a consultant gynaecologist friend of mine rightly puts it, endometriosis is like grass growing beyond the garden, out on the stone path as well.

Although the endometrium looks bulky its tissue is fragile and delicate, like candy floss or cotton wool, and can float around easily. Sometimes small pieces of endometrial tissue break away and float backwards or upwards through the Fallopian tubes into the abdominal cavity, settling on whatever tissue they meet first. Patches are often found in the small pouch area behind the uterus, on the ovaries or on the intestines. Occasionally, tiny fragments of the endometrium can travel through the blood or lymphatic system to the lungs and brain, and the distinct brown patches are instantly recognized by experienced surgeons.

This condition occurs in 3–10 per cent of women of reproductive age, and is a cause of infertility in about 30–40 per cent of cases.

## Symptoms

For some women the first they are aware of any stray endometrial growths is when the rogue patches are discovered during unrelated surgery or an abdominal exploration investigating problems with conceiving. A common symptom, however, is pelvic pain, especially before the start of a period. It is believed that these endometrial deposits continue to respond to the hormonal cycles as if they were still in the womb, and just before a period they swell and cause pain.

Endometriosis can also cause some spotting before your periods or in between them. This is not heavy bleeding, but is very uncomfortable and irritating.

Endometrial patches can also cause pain when they land on the intestines. They slowly grow and stick neighbouring sections of intestines together. These patches are termed adhesions and are the most common complication of endometriosis. When this happens the flow of gas or digested waste through the intestines becomes restricted, resulting in bloating and pain. Should endometrial patches spread aggressively they can block the intestines or urinary tract.

Although endometriosis and infertility are frequently linked, the exact relationship between the two is not understood, since deposits rarely block the uterine tubes. It is possible that such breaking away indicates that the endometrium is flaky and fragile, and so not healthy enough to facilitate implantation of a fertilized egg.

## Causes

The cause of endometriosis is not known precisely. Because doctors can't provide a cause for their patients, confusion abounds. Very often, women read about the symptoms and nature of endometriosis and liken the condition to cancer, because it spreads from its original site to other organs. This is incorrect, but it frequently adds another worry to period pains, the prospect of being infertile, the complications of drug therapy and so on.

## Treatment to relieve pain

*Diet:*

In my opinion a number of factors contribute to the pain, as no single reason can satisfy the criteria. Mechanical reason is the most logical explanation. Abdominal gas tends to increase premenstrually due to pelvic congestion (increased blood flow to the pelvic area). This extra fluid applies pressure on the walls of the rectum and 'flattens' it, obstructing the passage of wind or gas that is formed routinely in the intestines and habitually eliminated. This gas can build up and later stretch the abdominal wall, which leads to pain in the tendons attached to the pubic bone.

Reducing gas formation helps reduce such pain, so cut out from your diet anything that encourages

# DR ALI'S POINTS

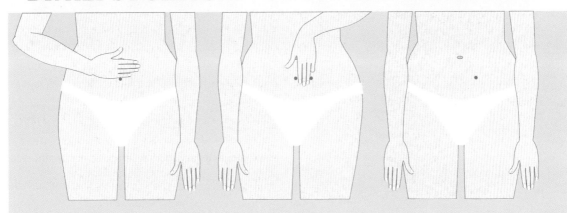

After years of prodding abdominal walls searching for trigger points to alleviate abdominal pain, I discovered two distinct small areas in the lower abdomen that do exactly that.

◆ Measure four fingers down from the navel and three to four fingers across to the left or right, you'll come across a dip – there's one on each side. You can sink your index finger slightly into the abdominal wall. One or both these points will be unusually sore to touch before your periods when there is generalized pain on the corresponding side (or both sides) of the abdomen. The soreness is so distinct that if you move just a few millimetres away from the dip, it cannot be felt.

◆ The straight muscles of the abdomen taper down into tendons that are ultimately attached to the pubic bone. At the point where the straight muscles begin to taper, there is reduced firmness of the abdominal wall. The dips either side are at these points. My belief is that the ring formed by muscles at this point is the point at which a small hernia may occur when there is excessive gas in the abdomen. The peritoneum (the protective sac enclosing the abdominal organs) protrudes into this soft area and causes irritation around the rim of the ring. That is why it is sore to touch.

◆ Massage the rim of this ring for a minute or so, with your index finger, and the soreness disappears. So does the abdominal pain. You'll be surprised how effective this treatment is.

abdominal gas. The worst dietary culprits are:

◆ fizzy drinks
◆ vegetables and cereals high in insoluble fibre (roughage), such as brassicas and bran
◆ dried beans and lentils
◆ radishes
◆ yeast products (including bread and beer) and excess sugar, which encourage fermentation in the gut

◆ Don't cut fibre out of your diet completely, as it is vital for a healthy digestion; just avoid the more fibrous parts, such as broccoli stalks.

*Other forms of pain relief:*
Colicky pains (which come and go in waves) can be treated with acupuncture or homeopathy (use 2–3 drops of belladonna tincture in water) or with anti-spasmodic drugs (ask your physician).

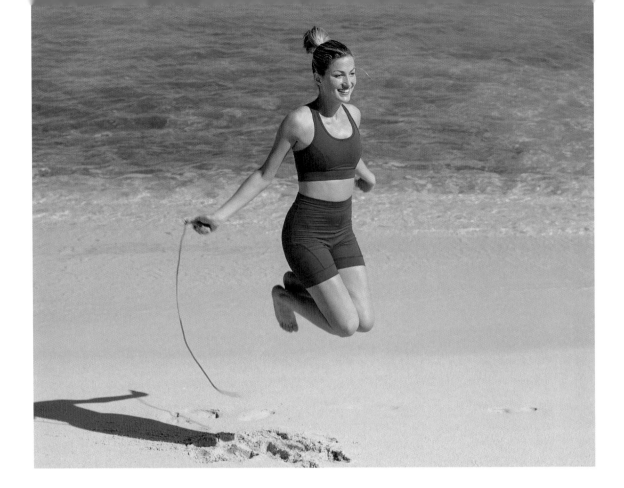

A continuous and unabating pain, which might be dull or severe, is very effectively eased by a specific form of massage (see box on page 105). I use this to treat any generalized abdominal pain.

**Treatment to curtail the spread:**

Whenever the cause of a disease or condition is not known, a general treatment to improve the well-being and self-regulation of the body's functions is always recommended. Lifestyle therapy, incorporating neck massage and specific therapeutic yoga keeps the body's functions on track (see Lifestyle Programme).

The endometrium responds to female hormones (it no longer becomes a problem after the menopause), so conventional medical treatment is to counteract oestrogen levels with androgens. However, this can be quite drastic: a drop in oestrogen levels can lead to osteoporosis and periods may stop, and hair growth on the face can be an embarrassing symptom.

Instead, I often recommend a high-protein diet and vigorous muscle-building exercises. The more muscle you build up, the less endometriosis seems to spread – perhaps because the steroids that muscle-bulk building releases into the system are only similar to androgens. They are not literally androgens, and do not bear any other qualities that could cause, for example, hirsutism. Instead of taking hormones to relieve pain, exercises should be given preference.

*Supplements:*
- zinc (linked to regulating hormonal functions).
- shilajit, a bitumen-like rock found in the Himalayas. This is rich in magnesium, zinc and other minerals. It is used traditionally to regulate hormonal functions (male monkeys – and, legend has it, dragons – licked this mineral compound before mating). Using this for endometriosis helps to regulate the spread of this potentially aggressive condition.

# Polycystic ovary syndrome
## (PCOS)

As the name suggests, this is not a single disease but a syndrome, i.e. a combination of symptoms that occur together. PCOS is characterized by:

◆ menstrual irregularities (usually lack of periods)
◆ infertility
◆ obesity
◆ hirsutism
◆ insulin resistance.

### Causes

Exactly why multiple cysts develop in the ovaries is not known, but their presence explains this varied collection of symptoms.

When some follicles in an ovary become filled with fluid and enlarge to form cysts (follicle stimulating hormone or FSH may be responsible for this abnormal ballooning), the eggs in these cysts disappear. The ovaries themselves become bulky and inactive, and healthy follicles do not function very well either, perhaps because they are squashed by neighbouring cysts. Fertility drops.

The ovaries produce and are influenced by several hormones. Although it may seem odd, some of these are androgens, the male hormones. For example, the stroma, which nourishes the egg follicles, secretes androgens as well as oestrogen. Normally, these male hormones are converted in the ovaries to oestrogen, but in PCOS this does not happen – again, perhaps the large cysts squashing the healthy ovarian tissue impair its normal function. The result is an excess of androgens (including testosterone). Their presence upsets the balance in a female body, causing periods to stop and increased hair growth on the face.

Obesity linked to PCOS is also hormone-related. The hypothalamus, which controls hormone release, is the home of the appetite centre. If the hypothalamus is not functioning well because of a reduced blood supply, then the glucose supply (via blood) to the appetite centre is also less. The appetite centre responds by creating a demand for food, which often manifests itself as a craving for something sweet. However, not all the fat of women with PCOS is associated with overeating. White fat (cellulite) is not dietary in origin but is a by-product of a defensive mechanism of the body. The reaction to an overload of male hormones is to convert them to a 'safe' form similar to oestrogen and then store this excess as white fat. (There is more on this in the chapter on Weight Control.)

With PCOS there is also increased insulin production (which can be tested), leading to insulin-resistant diabetes. Diabetes is linked to obesity and the increased insulin production helps androgen levels to rise.

## STRESS MANAGEMENT

PCOS is a worrying and upsetting condition because it seems to hit at the very heart of your femininity: male-pattern hair growth, a body too fat to be attractive, the threat of infertility. It is important to remain calm and keep a sense of proportion: this is not your fault, it is just a condition that you have. The advice below can help. Allowing stress to dominate can only do further harm – see Infertility, page 116 – so take stress management seriously. Meditation and relaxation techniques (see pages 73–4) are useful, and the regular massage sessions recommended below are calming and mood-enhancing.

**Treatments**

When cysts are large and cause pain or bear the risk of rupture, then surgery is usually recommended. The use of the contraceptive pill is often effective in regulating the periods.

*For losing weight:*

Conventional doctors usually suggest that overweight is the root cause of the problem, and that losing weight will allow menstruation to return to normal, and with it, hopefully, fertility. However, because white fat is not food-related, even a strict diet and exercise regime fails to reduce much weight, and this can be very frustrating. If depression with your disorder leads to comfort eating, this can compound the problem.

For my advice on overcoming this frustrating condition, see Conquering Hormonal Weight Gain, page 240.

Physical activity is important for reducing weight and for general health, but don't take up a very vigorous exercise regime. Lifting weights and other muscle-building or highly aggressive forms of exercise can make the situation worse by increasing the level of androgens and other masculine-style hormones. Choose gentle but therapeutic forms of exercise such as yoga, tai chi, walking or swimming (see Lifestyle Programme).

*For improving hormonal function:*

Neck and shoulder massage, combined with yoga as described in the Lifestyle Programme, are highly beneficial. Osteopathy, cranial osteopathy, chiropractic and forms of deep tissue massage are very effective for improving blood flow to the brain.

Improving the blood flow to the pituitary–hypothalamic area of the brain is helpful in PCOS in several ways.

◆ On a signal from the hypothalamus, the pituitary secretes follicle-stimulating hormones and luteinizing hormones, which are instrumental in the function of the ovaries (see page 88). When these parts of the brain are performing well they help the ovaries, and in turn the uterus, to function well too.
◆ The pituitary regulates the functions of the adrenal glands, which are a source of androgens. With androgen levels better controlled, facial hair and hormonal weight gain can improve and there is more chance of improving the ovarian follicles.
◆ The pituitary also regulates the thyroid gland, which often get affected with PCOS.
◆ Keeping the appetite centre in the hypothalamus well supplied with glucose via a good blood supply satisfies its demand and reduces food cravings, which can of course contribute significantly to weight loss.
◆ The hypothalamus also includes the centre controlling water retention. If this is not functioning well the result can be fluid retention, adding to weight problems.

*To counteract the effect of androgens:*

◆ aloe vera capsules: 1 capsule twice daily for six months
◆ include in your diet: rhubarb, yam, soya products, coriander leaves
◆ almonds: these mimic the effect of oestrogens and annul the harsh effect of androgens. Soak them for 24 hours before eating.

*Supplements:*

◆ I generally use homeopathic remedies for the control of multiple cysts; consult a qualified homeopath for the best suited to you. I often recommend pulsatilla 30: 2 tablets three times a day for three days around mid-cycle, or mid-calendar month (if your periods have stopped).

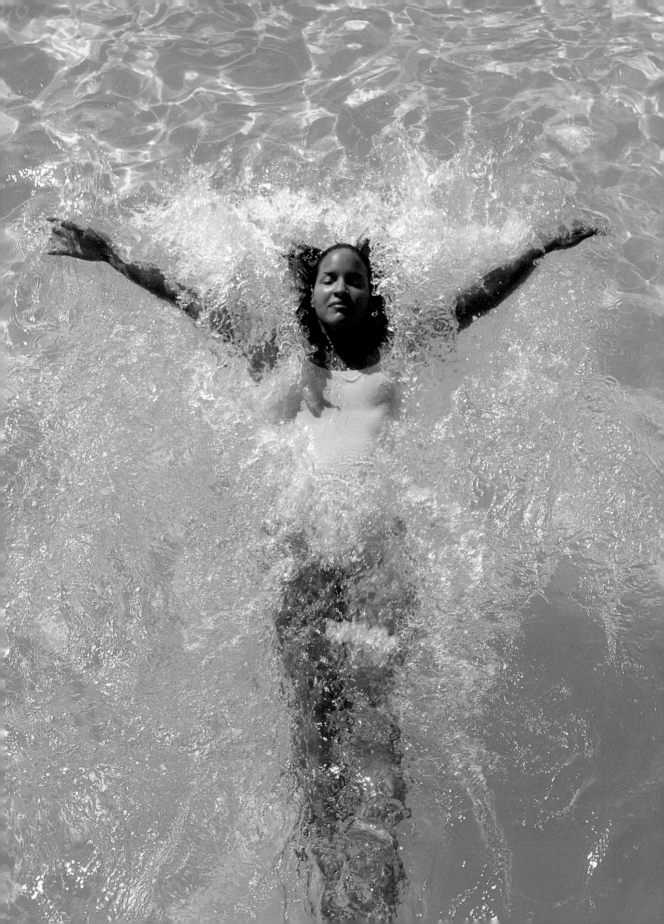

# Fibroids

These are benign growths in the muscle layer of the uterus. Although the label 'fibroids' is often used as a general term, they are actually part of a group of benign tumours called leiomyomas. Growths consisting of more fibre or connective tissue (ligaments or collagen fibres) than muscle are fibroids; growths with equal fibre and muscle content are called fibromyomas; and muscle-only growths are called myomas.

About 25 per cent of all women of reproductive age have leiomyomas in one form or another (they are more common in women of African or Afro-Caribbean origin), but many are unaware of them. They usually appear in clusters of spherical nodules, clearly demarcated from the surrounding uterine muscle tissue. Mostly they are small in size, but have been known to reach vast proportions. (In a remote area of India, I once arranged the surgery of a woman who had a swelling like a full-term pregnancy. She had endured the discomfort of this condition for five years as there was no local medical help.)

## Cause

The exact cause of leiomyomas is not known but oestrogen is often implicated – oestrogen (as an ingredient in contraceptive pills) and pregnancy can increase their size and they usually shrink away with the menopause, when oestrogen levels drop. They can similarly shrink after pregnancy.

## Symptoms

Although they originate from muscle fibres, fibroids and their like don't function like muscles, but their presence can be a hindrance. When the uterine muscles contract or go into spasm during muscular cramps, for example, they can make the pain worse. They may cause the endometrium to bleed more during periods or between cycles and they may make it more difficult for a fertilized egg to implant itself in the uterus.

Larger growths can cause backache as they press on nerves, heaviness in the pelvic region, make intercourse painful and cause urinary problems, constipation and even prolapse. They can trigger a spontaneous abortion.

Leiomyomas can shrink, liquefy and become cysts or harden and turn septic, or they may stop developing and become totally inert but not disappear. Rarely (in less than 0.5 per cent of cases) they can become malignant (leiomyosarcomas).

## Treatments

There are various types of treatment available. First, the rate of growth should be established by six-monthly ultrasound or manual examinations. If there are no symptoms and little visible swelling, then no intervention is necessary. A rapidly growing tumour should be kept under observation, to prevent it leading to complications.

Removal of small fibroids by keyhole surgery is helpful if it is suspected that they have been preventing conception. As a routine precautionary measure, the excised tissue will be examined in a laboratory to make sure there are no signs of malignancy.

There are drugs that suppress or neutralize the stimulation of oestrogen and progesterone by the ovaries. This treatment will cause the growths to shrink to about half their size, but there are side-effects. Blocking the hormones in this way creates, in effect, an artificial and premature menopause: periods will stop, and there may be hot flushes and other menopausal symptoms. If continued for over six months, there may be an increased risk of osteoporosis. Sometimes, if a hysterectomy is necessary, this form of chemical shrinkage beforehand may make it possible for the operation to be a vaginal hysterectomy, rather than the more major abdominal operation (see page 112).

Emolization is a popular method of treatment. This involves chemically blocking the uterine artery, cutting off the blood supply to the growths. Without blood to nourish them, they shrink and degenerate.

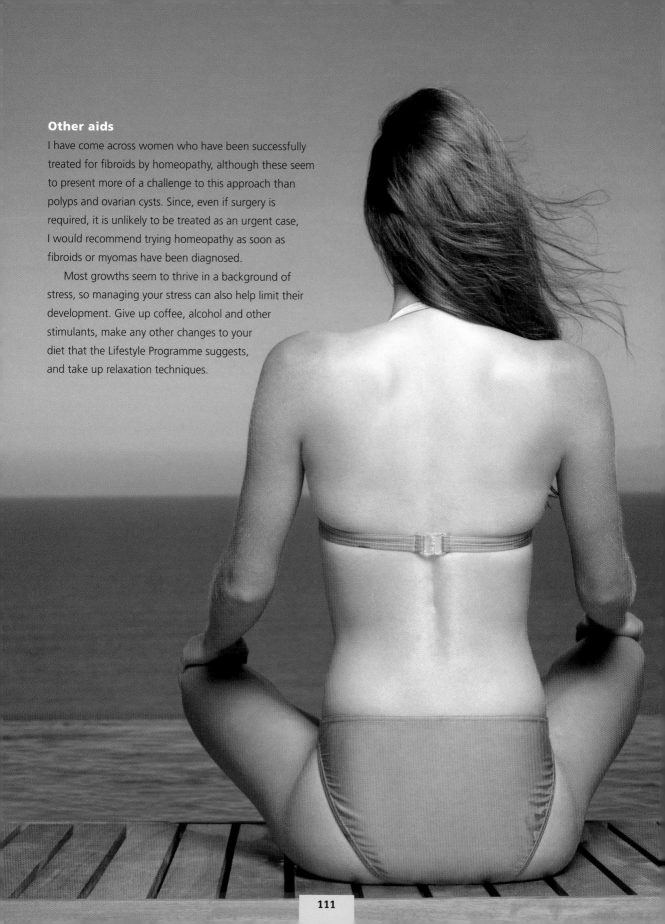

## Other aids

I have come across women who have been successfully treated for fibroids by homeopathy, although these seem to present more of a challenge to this approach than polyps and ovarian cysts. Since, even if surgery is required, it is unlikely to be treated as an urgent case, I would recommend trying homeopathy as soon as fibroids or myomas have been diagnosed.

Most growths seem to thrive in a background of stress, so managing your stress can also help limit their development. Give up coffee, alcohol and other stimulants, make any other changes to your diet that the Lifestyle Programme suggests, and take up relaxation techniques.

# Hysterectomy

Hysterectomy is the complete removal of the uterus. Until comparatively recently, it was an almost routine operation, seen as a cure for all manner of 'female' complaints. Although it is the second most common operation performed on women, it is now performed much less often as women have questioned its necessity. Newer technologies are also providing alternatives.

The most pressing reason for a hysterectomy is cancer in the uterus or cervix. It may also be recommended for other severe conditions that have not responded to previous treatments. These conditions may include:

◆ heavy bleeding and pain due to fibroids. A hysterectomy should not be necessary for even quite large fibroids that do not cause severe pain or bleeding. After the menopause, they are likely to shrink and disappear of their own accord.
◆ a uterus that is rapidly swelling from bulky fibroids or a growing myometrium.
◆ benign tumours, especially when growing into the cavity of the uterus.
◆ abnormal bleeding and pressure in the pelvis, perhaps causing permanent incontinence and bladder problems.
◆ severe menstrual pains leading to fainting and illness every month.
◆ prolapse of uterus (see page 217).
◆ abscess, pelvic inflammatory disease, severe leucorrhoea (white or yellow smelly discharge from uterus), when antibiotics or anti-inflammatories have not worked.

## IS IT NECESSARY?

There are plenty of reasons to question whether a hysterectomy is necessary. This is a radical operation, and there is risk attached to any such procedure. The uterus is only a small organ, but it has a tremendous effect on your body. An oophorectomy involves the removal of the ovaries as well as the uterus: the procedure must be discussed beforehand, as removal of both has the effect of inducing an instant menopause (due to the loss of hormones produced by the ovaries), which, if very premature, may have long-term consequences for your general health. For a younger woman, there can be deep-seated psychological effects of having the uterus removed. You will not technically be any less 'complete' a woman, but many feel exactly this, and the irredeemable loss of the ability to bear children may be difficult to come to terms with.

Some hospitals, and some surgeons, will turn to hysterectomy as the answer more readily than others. Do not hurriedly agree to a hysterectomy because of pain. Ensure that other conditions, such as intestinal adhesions, gall stones, kidney stones and even appendicitis, all of which can cause severe pain in the abdomen, have been ruled out. If there is a pelvic mass that cannot be evaluated, an ultrasound scan and an MRI scan should help diagnosis before surgery is considered.

That said, a hysterectomy can sometimes be the only answer, and may be life-saving. Discuss with your doctor or gynaecologist the possibility of a vaginal, rather than abdominal operation. Using the vagina to gain access to the uterus rather than cutting into the pelvic area lessens the trauma to the body generally, and reduces the chance of infection. In cases of cancer, however, it will probably be necessary to remove the ovaries too, and it will be important to examine lymph nodes in the pelvic region for any signs of the cancer having spread. This will probably require abdominal surgery.

## BEFORE SURGERY

Any operation is debilitating, and you will recover more quickly and more completely if you can prepare your body as well as possible beforehand (see page 278). Surgery on any part of the abdomen will leave the whole area feeling sore. Any pain will be exacerbated by additional pressure from abdominal gas or blocked bowels.

◆ Make sure you do not have high stomach acid. Heartburn and indigestion will seem all the more acute after abdominal surgery. Gastritis also impairs iron absorption. Eat slowly and avoid citrus fruits, deep-fried foods, alcohol (except an occasional glass of wine or drakshasava (an ayurvedic balsam of fermented grapes and herbs), painkillers (unless there is severe menstrual pain), high doses of vitamin C (more than 500g at a time), nuts, chillies, heavy curries, pineapple and mango.
◆ Make sure you are not constipated.

If one of your symptoms has been heavy bleeding, you may be anaemic to some degree.

◆ Eat plenty of foods rich in iron and in elements that aid iron absorption: liver, red meat, game, pulses, dark green leafy vegetables, dried ginger.
◆ Take iron supplements.

Prepare yourself for after the operation.

◆ You will not be able to be very active for a few weeks afterwards, and this and the hormonal changes mean you are likely to put on weight. Without depriving yourself of any nutrition, lose what excess weight you can now. See the chapter on Weight Control.

## SEE ALSO...

As I said at the very beginning of this chapter, reproductive health is not independent of the rest of the body. Other sections of this book that may be relevant or helpful include: Ectopic pregnancy (page 147), Miscarriage (page 171), Contraception (page 132), Menopause (page 302), Weight Control (page 219).

◆ Yoga and relaxation techniques will help to still your mind and improve your well-being. You may react to losing your uterus more strongly than you think.

## AFTER SURGERY

◆ Follow the recuperation guidance in the chapter on General Disorders and Problems. Pay particular attention to what you eat and drink, because your whole abdominal area will be tender and vulnerable, so your digestive system should not be put under any strain.
◆ To help ward off weight gain, keep carbohydrate, alcohol and fat intake under control once you are eating proper meals again.
◆ Take hormone support supplements for three to six months to regulate the hormones.

# Infertility

About 90 per cent of couples having unprotected intercourse will conceive within a year. If a couple trying for a baby do not succeed in conceiving after this time then infertility becomes a concern.

The longer the infertility continues, the more frustrated a couple can become. Friends conceiving without apparent difficulty seem like a mute reproach; even the sight of children with their parents can bring on tears, and insensitive hints about 'the patter of tiny feet' can add to the anguish. Each partner starts to blame the other, libido drops, and the whole relationship can be endangered by a range of psychological reactions, including denial, guilt, repression and loss of self-esteem. In certain cultures, the threat of being cast aside in favour of a fertile woman can add to the desperation. Stress levels soar. And, as we shall see, stress can actually inhibit conception.

Infertility is not the same as sterility, which is a complete inability to conceive. Sterility in women may have several causes, such as an unnaturally small uterus, hormonal problems, lack of ovulation or a major ovarian disorder, and these possibilities should be investigated so that they can be ruled out or treated. Infertility is simply the decrease in ability to conceive – it is not a disease or a syndrome, but a condition or a situation. There are no symptoms, and sometimes no cause can be found. The only way of knowing that a particular treatment is working or not is when a baby is conceived.

## Checking out possible causes

Several physical conditions inhibit conception, mostly relating either to a hormonal problem or a physical impediment such as polycystic ovaries or endometriosis. Here are some of the things your doctor may look for.

### INDICATIONS OF OVULATION

Perfect coordination is paramount: if ovulation does not take place, there will be no egg to fertilize, and if the lining of the uterus is not prepared to receive a fertilized egg, there will be no pregnancy. By using ultrasound it is possible to see if there is a matured egg cell (larger than the rest) developed in one or other ovary. Ovulation can also be detected by taking the basal body temperature (BBT) early in the morning, when body temperature is naturally at its lowest. A sudden drop then rise in temperature (due to a hormonal surge) indicates ovulation. This needs the use of a special fertility thermometer.

Progesterone, secreted in the second half of the monthly cycle, changes the quality and quantity of mucus secreted by the cervix. This mucus may be discharged into the vagina soon after ovulation. It is distinct from regular discharge, and has been described as glutinous, like egg white.

Polycystic ovaries (see page 107), ovarian disease or hormonal messages failing to trigger the right responses at the right time can all impede or prevent ovulation.

## HORMONAL IMBALANCE

Any upset to the delicate balance and sequence of hormonal levels can inhibit conception. A high level of milk-producing hormone (prolactin), for example, can suppress ovulation and even periods (which is why women breastfeeding are unlikely to conceive). Certain drugs, including the contraceptive pill, can cause a rise in prolactin. Too high a level of androgens (male hormones) will also result in problems.

If not caused by thyroid or liver disease (the liver metabolizes oestrogen), then a hormonal imbalance is probably due to a malfunction or under-performance within the pituitary or hypothalamus, which coordinate hormonal production. The reason for this might be a congenital problem or a tumour, but more often is explained by a trauma to the neck or head (whiplash or a fall), or repetitive strain or tension, impeding blood flow to this area of the brain – for more on the effects of this, see page 240. See also obesity, below.

## UTERINE CONDITIONS

A menstrual flow that is good and lasts for four or five days indicates that the lining of the uterus (endometrium) developing each month is thick enough for implantation to occur. A poor-quality endometrium will not be able to sustain a fertilized egg. The thickness of the endometrium can be measured by ultrasound.

Fibroids, endometriosis (see page 104–6) or a uterine infection can also prevent an egg from implanting itself in the uterus.

## HEALTHY SPERM

A common cause of non-conception is the failure of sperm to fertilize an egg. Reasons for this include:

- low sperm count
- poor motility (sluggish sperm)
- low testosterone; pituitary or hypothalamic malfunction
- impotence or impaired sperm production

These can all be tested and should be ruled out before looking further.

## OBESITY

If you are very overweight, this is frequently quickly diagnosed as the cause. It may at first seem an odd link, as many very large women also get pregnant without problems. However, as the chapter on Weight Control explains, obesity can have several causes.

Both yellow and white fat contribute to obesity, but white fat (cellulite) builds up because of an excess of androgens (male hormones) which are being converted into oesterone (similar to oestrogen and so acceptable to a female body) and stored as cellulite. Excess female hormones are similarly stored. So obesity that is predominantly white fat indicates a hormonal imbalance. Polycystic ovaries and adrenal problems can be at the root of this.

The hormone leptin, which is synthesized by fat cells, has also been blamed for suppressing ovulation.

## Stress

There is one contributory factor towards infertility that I have not yet mentioned: stress. Not every woman you might classify as highly strung, driven or overworked has difficulty becoming pregnant, but the role stress plays in inhibiting conception is widely recognized. There are many anecdotal examples:

■ Many couples who adopt often subsequently bear children naturally. Once the stresses of deadlines, guilt, dilemma and pressure on relationships are taken away, conception often becomes much easier.

■ At the time that East Pakistan was liberated to become independent Bangladesh, I happened to do some volunteer work with the refugees near Calcutta. Many women reported being raped by soldiers. A doctor working with the refugees said that although thousands were raped, only 200 or so were reported to be pregnant as a consequence. Considering that a woman can conceive for approximately a quarter of each month, the figure should have been higher. Rape victims are less likely to get pregnant.

■ As a result of an article in the *Daily Mail* in 1998 featuring some of the mothers I had successfully helped with my method of management of infertility, hundreds of women and couples came to see me. Most had no known cause of infertility, but over 60 per cent were highly stressed and had highly demanding jobs.

To some extent the effects of stress are measurable. A consultant gynaecologist friend of mine told me that while doing ultrasonic examinations of the uterus, the slightest pinprick stimulation of the skin caused immediate contraction of the uterine muscles. Physical or emotional pain does affect our involuntary muscles. Just as stress increases the heartbeat and constricts blood vessels, so the involuntary uterine and Fallopian tube muscles can also contract due to physical or emotional stress. Both these conditions can be detrimental for conception.

Moreover, stress hormones are similar in character to androgens (male hormones), which may explain why putting the body under excessive physical and well as psychological stress – hard training programmes, long hours without sleep – seems to decrease fertility.

It is sadly ironic that stress can be a barrier to successful conception, and failing to conceive often increases stress levels.

## Treatments

There are a number of treatments available for infertility, from drugs and surgery to IVF and egg donation, but success is variable. If failure follows failure, it is easy to get caught up in a desperate chase, trying one treatment after another after another. The strain, both financial and on your sense of proportion and your relationship, can be very damaging. When treatments don't work doctors and practitioners are bombarded with sometimes unanswerable questions, they bear the brunt of a couple's frustrations and can be verbally attacked. Quite naturally, they often become cautious and reluctant to offer further treatment.

My belief, especially if no obvious cause has been discovered, is that you should give Mother Nature, via your innate healing power, a chance before you embark on any invasive treatment. Reproduction, like breathing, digestion or circulation, is a basic feature of human life, so laying down conditions that lead to self-rectification of any infertility problems is very important.

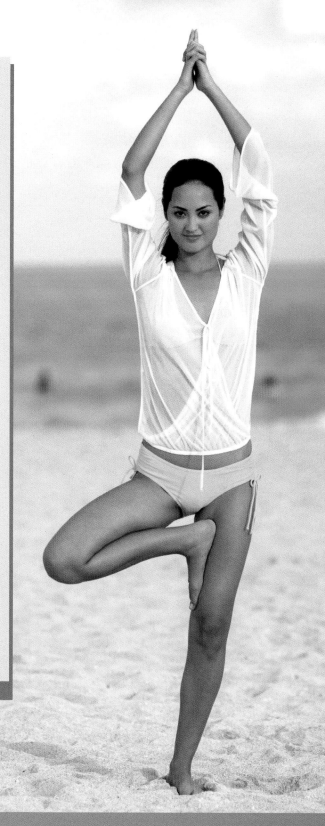

## CASE STUDY

# Stress: block to a natural phenomenon

Verona came to seem me when she was 36 and had been trying to get pregnant for three years. She was against IVF, as she was worried about side-effects of fertility drugs.

She had a regular 28-day menstrual cycle and normal periods lasting four days. When talking to her, I realized that there was nothing wrong other than a stressful job and home life. I changed her diet (to put less strain on her body), gave her neck and shoulder massages twice a month and taught her some relaxation breathing techniques. She also took up yoga and walking in the park. After three months of this simple treatment, she conceived, had a trouble-free pregnancy (maintaining her new regime) and gave birth easily to a baby girl.

Three years later, Verona came back. She had been trying to conceive a second child for six months, without success. Each failure left her more frustrated and she worried that, at almost 40, time was running out. I asked her to adopt the same lifestyle changes as before and, within a few months, she was pregnant. This time it was a boy.

Verona's case was mentioned, along with two others, in an article on my 'pregnancy secrets'. In fact, there is no secret. You have to listen to your body's requirements. Good nutrition, stress management and increased energy levels help to regulate the body's functions. Pregnancy is a natural phenomenon and should happen without effort.

## NUTRITION

Follow the general guidance for nutrition in the Lifestyle Programme, and in particular ...

Avoid anything that may cause digestive problems, as this can interfere with blood circulation in the abdomen:

◆ yeast products (bloating, gas)
◆ fried food (acidity)
◆ excess chillies, garlic and spices (acidity)
◆ blue cheese (e.g. Stilton), mushrooms (gas)
◆ excess sugar (which will feed yeasts and fungi)
◆ canned products (preservatives, excess sugar/salt)
◆ coffee, excess salt, alcohol (irritants)
◆ fizzy water (gas).

Avoid any foods whose acidity may have spermicidal effects:

◆ citrus fruits
◆ vinegar and vinegary foods such as pickles and mayonnaise
◆ acidic fruit such as pineapple, tomatoes.

Have things that are good to eat:

◆ organic produce (to minimize the ingestion of any chemicals that may have adverse effects)
◆ oily fish (mackerel, salmon, tuna, king fish, sardines, pilchards, etc; these contain vitamins E, A and D)
◆ calf's liver
◆ free-range eggs
◆ fish roe. Caviar is considered to be a potent aid to fertility as it contains fine and easily digestible protein (in Russia, in the days before most of their caviar was exported, it was eaten during pregnancy and breastfeeding), but it is extremely salty. Other roe, such as herring, is a good source of nourishment but without the excess salt
◆ almonds (soaked for 24 hours to soften them), pistachios, walnuts, Brazil nuts and hazelnuts contain zinc, useful for fertility
◆ spinach, okra, mint and basil leaves, pears, red apples, carrots, grapes, cherries. In general include plenty of green vegetables and non-acidic fruit in your diet
◆ pomegranate juice or the fruit itself. This aids blood synthesis and helps to improve uterine functions; it is a traditional remedy to improve fertility.

## MASSAGE

The neck and shoulder massage techniques described in the Lifestyle Programme are beneficial on several levels:

◆ improving blood flow to the pituitary–hypothalamic area helps with their functions of controlling reproductive hormones
◆ relieving stress
◆ improving sleep and increasing energy
◆ enhancing mood and the 'feel-good' factor.

All these help the entire body and improve the chances of conceiving naturally. In particular, have a massage at least two days before and one day after ovulation. Involving your partner in regular massage sessions (and you can return the favour) also heightens sensuality and bonding. Massaging shortly before bedtime induces a good sleep, which will enhance in both of you a 'feel-good' factor for lovemaking in the early morning.

## RELAXATION

Have lukewarm showers, rather than a hot bath at night. Although a hot bath is relaxing, it interferes with the blood circulation. Your body temperature rises considerably while you are in the water, and as soon as you come out you lose heat quickly, and your body is easily chilled. Hot baths can also dilate the uterus – indeed an old-fashioned method of self-abortion was to consume a heavy dose of alcohol while sitting in a hot bath with salt and mustard in the water to help increase body temperature and dilate involuntary muscles, including the uterine muscles.

## EXERCISE

Exercise is important for general health and a sense of well-being, but avoid vigorous exercise that increases muscle bulk. The hormones that are released by such muscle-building are similar to male hormones and could upset the hormonal balance vital to conception. Swimming, walking and gentle rhythmic exercises are all good, and I particularly recommend yoga and tai chi.

## SUPPLEMENTS

Do not take too many vitamins and supplements as they may interfere with the body's delicate system during this period.

◆ shatavari: one tablet twice daily for ten days from the end of your period (i.e. stopping just before ovulation).
◆ aloe vera capsules (freeze dried): as for shatavari.
◆ mix a few (4–5) saffron strands with honey and milk and have this daily.

Homeopathy, Chinese herbal treatment, acupuncture and spiritual healing have all worked for some women.

## Breathing exercise

The breathing techniques that are part of therapeutic yoga are especially advantageous, as they invigorate the body with increased oxygen uptake as well as calm the nervous system. Do the three exercises described in the Lifestyle Programme (see Controlled breathing, pages 73–4) every day, repeating each 10–15 times.

Bellowing your abdomen out during inhalation and sucking it in during exhalation is exactly the opposite of what most people do, but is worth practising.

Once you have mastered the technique it is a powerful method of stress relief and relaxation. It also benefits the abdominal organs. While bellowed out, the abdomen creates negative pressure in the abdominal cavity and so the diaphragm flattens out and moves downwards, and the blood rushes in to all parts of the abdomen. When the abdomen is sucked in, the diaphragm domes and the venous blood from the internal organs is pushed out.

# Conception day

The egg can live for up to 72 hours after ovulation while ejaculated sperm cells can live for a maximum of 120 hours (usually less). Statistics show that the most fertile period is 48 hours (two days) before ovulation. After ovulation, the chances drop rapidly. Isolated pregnancies happen to have taken place earlier than 72 hours before and up to four days after.

The following is some practical advice to optimize the chances of conception.

◆ Abstain from lovemaking for a week before, then make love one day before and on the day of expected ovulation.

◆ The optimum time to make love is in the early hours of the morning (around 5 or 6 a.m.). Although the actual ovulation can take place at any time of day, it is most likely to take place in the early hours of the morning (around 4 a.m.) as the body prepares for waking up.

◆ Go to bed early the previous night and get a good night's sleep.

◆ Do not rush or panic. Take your time.

◆ Put a pillow under your hips to prevent any spilling or wastage of sperm from your vagina, and stay lying on your back like that for at least half an hour (go to the toilet before lovemaking so that you don't have to worry about a full bladder).

◆ Lie in bed for a couple of hours more to rest. Maintain your sense of calm (meditation and peaceful music can help).

This does, however, make several assumptions: that you can detect ovulation (either by noticing a change in vaginal mucus or feeling a change in temperature) and that your ovulation cycle is regular (which it might not be, even if your periods are). It is a matter of knowing your own body and learning its rhythms. It is also worth remembering that even a regular cycle can be affected by all sorts of things, such as stress or long-haul travel, and its indicators masked by illness or medication, etc.

## IMPROVING SPERM PRODUCTION

Of course, men cannot be left out of this equation. In addition to participating in massage and other relaxing techniques, I recommend the following to improve sperm production:

◆ Egg flip: beat a raw egg (ensure it is very fresh and from a reputable supplier) into a glass of warm milk, stir thoroughly and add salt and pepper to taste. Have this at breakfast every day for seven days before your partner's ovulation time.

◆ Eat lean red meat and game. Every other day cook up some meat in a mixture of 'heating' flavourings and spices: garlic, ginger, onions, cloves, asafoetida, cardamom, cinnamon, saffron and olive oil. Cook on a slow heat and keep turning over. This heating and stirring helps energize or 'potentize' the meat by breaking up the fibres and makes them more readily digestible, so less energy is expended in digesting it.

◆ Take a match-head-sized piece of pure shilajit (available in some Indian grocery shops), mixed in warm milk and honey, every other day for a month. Shilajit is rich in magnesium, zinc and a host of minerals, and is considered a powerful aphrodisiac, stimulant to the immune system and energy booster.

Trying to follow a sometimes complicated regime to keep track of your most fertile days – noting when your period starts and when your vaginal mucus changes character, recording your rectal temperature, trying to decide whether or not that twinge was a sign of ovulation – can wreak havoc with your sex life. Do everything you can to avoid it becoming 'performing by numbers'– retaining the romance of lovemaking is very important (see the chapter on Sexual Health).

### TIPPING THE BALANCE IN YOUR FAVOUR

It is said that a woman may not conceive when she has a fever, bodily aches, backache, when depressed, extremely tired, suffering from palpitations, has fractures or wounds that are healing, experiences pain during coitus or fears penetration. While these are hardly contraceptive methods, for couples experiencing difficulty in conceiving, small things can sometimes tip the balance.

Personal hygiene is very important. Thrush or other infections and excessive vaginal discharge affect conditions in the vagina (see pages 214–15) and may have a spermicidal effect. Fungal foods such as mushrooms, bread, yeast spreads, beer and cheese, as well as anti-biotics, can also have spermicidal properties. If not kept scrupulously clean, a penis can harbour bacteria or fungi.

Tradition has it that the chances of conception are higher if the pleasure in lovemaking is great and the orgasms of the man and woman take place simultaneously or close to each other's. Thus, foreplay, love for each other, passion and deep arousal are very important for conception. Ancient literature suggests that couples that cannot conceive should learn the art of lovemaking.

Very frequent ejaculation weakens the quality of the sperm (it is said that from 40lb of food you get 1lb of flesh, from 40lb of flesh you get enough material for 1lb of blood, and 40lb of blood is equivalent to 1lb of sperm). The frequent loss of sperm needs to be backed by highly potent food and puts high demands on the male body to synthesize both blood and sperm.

Infertility is not a simple matter. It has to be approached sensibly and with patience.

## Technological aid

If a cause or significant contributory factor for your infertility has been diagnosed, drugs or surgery may be the answer. More radical measures are also available.

Artificial insemination (by partner or donor), surrogacy and egg donation are among the possibilities open to women who have not succeeded in conceiving, and there are several variations on in vitro fertilization (IVF), in which part of the process is carried out in a laboratory.

### WHAT IN VITRO FERTILIZATION (IVF) INVOLVES

The first stage is to be given drugs that can stimulate the ovarian follicles so that several eggs ovulate at once. These are then collected, fertilized with sperm cells in vitro (i.e. in a test tube), and the fertilized eggs allowed to develop before the best embryo is reintroduced into the womb. The process is carefully timed so that conditions for fertilization and implantation happen at the optimum moment. Because conditions are carefully controlled, the implantation success rate is quite high; the main problem is development and many pregnancies fail in the early stages.

Fertility clinics may try four cycles, but IVF exhausts the ovaries and it takes a while before they begin to function again. The drugs also have side-effects, such as bloating or making you highly agitated, but many women have felt it worth tolerating these and the personal intrusion in the hope of getting pregnant.

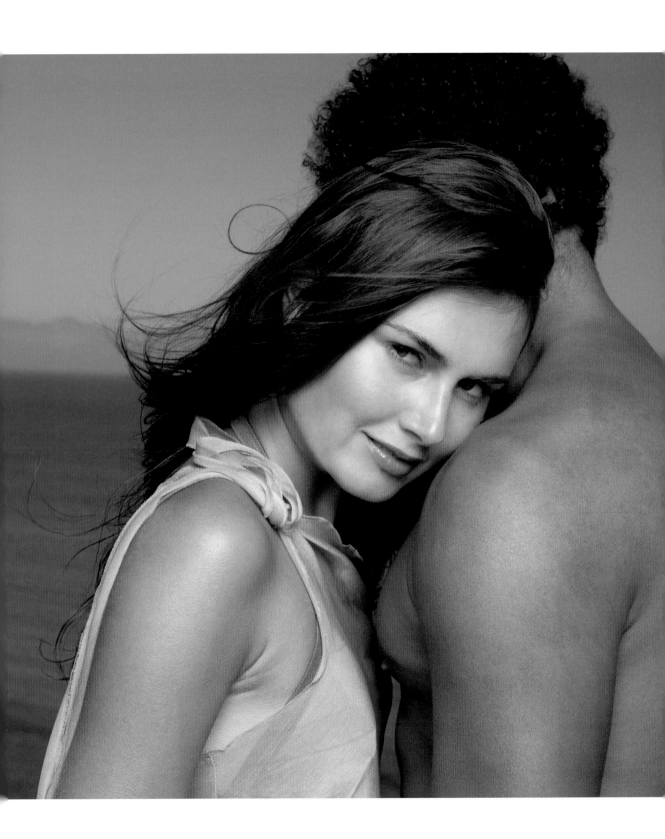

# chapter two

# sexual health

Sexual health ranges from protecting yourself from sexually transmitted infection or unwanted pregnancy to being fulfilled as a sexual being. This last subject could take up the whole book, but I shall limit myself here to a few specific points.

A healthy sex life is one of the most enjoyable aspects of life as a whole, and as such has immense benefits for your general health and well-being. If you do not intend to have children, you should be fully aware of the contraception options available, and if you have different sexual partners it's vital that you protect yourself against sexually transmitted infections.

# The power of sex

While men may go around boasting about 'male power' and masculine superiority, it is female sexual power that really dominates. The Hindu god Shiva's wife was Shakti, synonymous with universal power, and Mother Earth, or Mother Nature, or Gaia, are common expressions of that power. Kundalini, the 'female serpentine power' referred to in tantra yoga and meditative disciplines, is the supreme power that controls our life force.

Female sexuality is a deeply entwined blend of the physical and the mental. Just as poor health can affect a woman's sex life, a loss of libido, unfulfilled desire, painful sexual experience or the mental hurt of 'being used as a sex object' can cause deep psychological strain and affect a woman's whole health and well-being.

# Lovemaking
Making love with your partner is an essential part of a healthy relationship. The stimulation and relaxation that come through sex can be of great physical benefit to you both.

## Educating your partner

Women, for their own pleasure and satisfaction, should educate their partners. Sometimes men, even if sophisticated and intelligent in other ways, can be ignorant of a woman's needs or be very arrogant in matters of sex. Simply accepting the way he wants things can become an accepted rule, but can also be a real problem.

Both partners have to work together and participate in each other's enjoyment. Just as in eating, anticipating and preparation are themselves an appetite stimulant, and make the whole sexual encounter more pleasurable. Sounds, words, imagination and fantasy play as big a role in lovemaking as the physical act. Variety and experimentation give different flavours and pleasures just as recipes do to food. Learning what pleases each other leads to deeper and more fulfilling sexual encounters. This includes making an effort to look your best and creating a romantic mood as well as seeking out favourite erogenous zones.

On the more practical side:

■ The ideal time for making love is in the early hours of the morning, when you are both relaxed. (And a full bladder stimulates the nervous plexus, which controls dilation of blood vessels in the penis.)

■ It is said that sex should not be performed on a full stomach or when you are very hungry. A snack (fruits or nuts) helps to provide extra energy if you haven't eaten.

■ A little wine may help to relax the mind but it cannot compare to the sense of relaxation that massage, music, words and touch can bring. But excess alcohol interferes with the whole process.

■ Body odour and halitosis are very off-putting. Avoid foods that taint the breath. (Fish, for example, is good for you, but its smell on the breath is very unromantic.) Kadu and kariatu are traditional Indian herbal supplements that help to control abdominal gas.

■ Fit people are not necessarily better lovers, but they have the potential to be. Fatigue in the thighs, lower back, buttocks and abdomen reduces enjoyment and diverts your focus.

■ The more gentle the breathing, the more gentle the movements, the better the enjoyment. Hyperventilation comes with orgasm, but controlled breathing will retain or prolong climax (see Controlled breathing, pages 73–4).

■ Learning to focus your mind through yoga, pranayama (yogic breathing) and meditation, will help control and maintain calm.

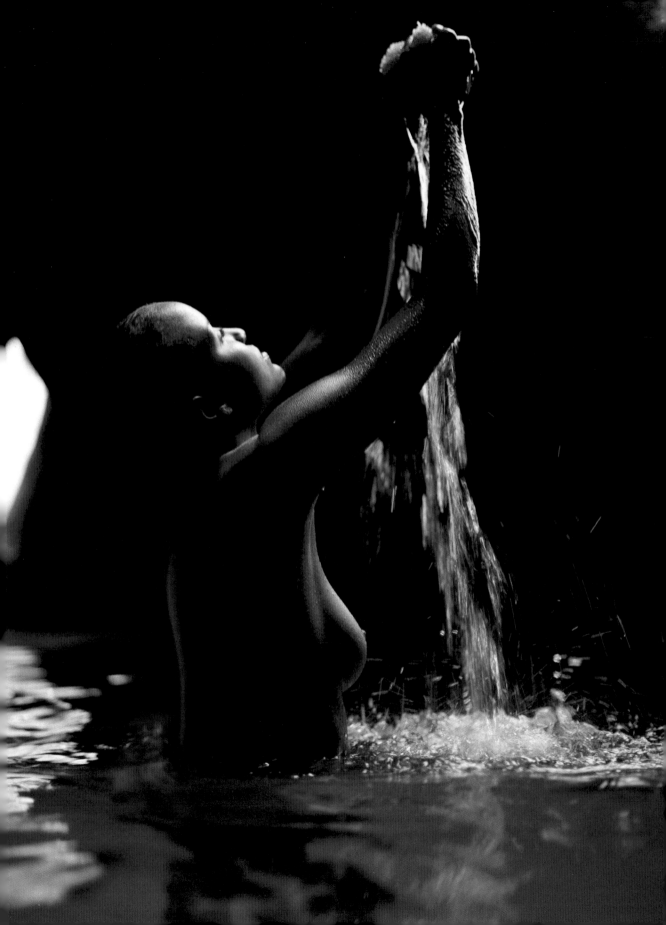

# Mind over body

The parts of the brain that control sexual desire and activities are the hypothalamus and limbic system. The hypothalamus is the highest centre of the autonomics or involuntary nervous system. The limbic system, located close by, is the centre for the emotions. Sexual desire is created in the hypothalamus (just as the desire to eat is), and then the message is sent to the limbic system to create the 'drive' and the actual physical act.

Although our muscles are under our voluntary control, much of what goes on during sexual intercourse, from vaginal lubrication to orgasm, involves the involuntary nervous system. But it is possible to influence these involuntary functions too.

It is believed that there are seven chakras or seats of energy in the body, the locations of which coincide with the distribution of the control centres of the involuntary nervous system. The cardiac chakra, for example, coincides with the collection of nerves controlling functions of the heart and lungs. Mooladhera, the lowest chakra or inguinal plexus, is the seat of kundalini, and controls bladder and bowel functions, sexual arousal, ejaculation and orgasm.

With different techniques it is possible to activate and control the involuntary nervous system. Control is easiest near the top of the body. Through the highest chakra, the pituitary–hypothalamus, you can mimic emotions: portray anger, imitate joy or shed false tears, quite easily. Control becomes progressively more difficult as you descend towards the lower parts of the body, but trained yogi can control their heart rate, aspects of their digestion and so on. To arouse kundalini, in the lowest part of the abdomen, takes great training and determination, which is why it has an aura of mystique and its very existence is questioned. Those who have mastered the art of channelling this energy can control many functions of body and mind, including clairvoyance, premonition, energy, sleep and orgasm.

## CASE STUDY

## Unexplained power surge

I have come across three female patients who, at the peak of orgasm, have experienced a feeling of lightning or great electrical force passing upwards from the base of the spinal column and passing out through the head. They saw a bright flash and occasionally heard a loud popping sound and felt a violent jerk, followed by a sense of euphoria. They were so terrified that they pushed their partners away and were left trembling and sweating. Psychiatrists they consulted could not understand this problem, and prescribed tranquillizers or anti-epileptic drugs. Having read books on kundalini and spoken to an old master of yoga, I have no doubt that these patients experienced spontaneous arousal of kundalini, without their mind or body being prepared.

Tantric meditation (see the chapter on Psychological Health), used to arouse kundalini, requires practice, perseverance, knowledge, patience and deep mutual understanding. When I hear of men going off to Hawaii for a two-week tantra course, I cannot but laugh. What a mockery of a sublime art!

There is no easy way of learning this sort of control over your sexual powers, no short cuts. However, the practice of yoga, breath control and meditation will help you to focus on and enhance your sexual performance.

# Loss or decrease in libido At some point in our lives most of us will experience a time when we lose interest in sex.

The hypothalamus, which controls sex drive, is a finely tuned part of the brain and therefore very sensitive. It is easily affected by fatigue, stress, worries, poor diet, poor blood flow to the brain and any number of sociological and psychological influences. Here are just some of the things that can cause you to lose interest in sex:

◆ stress from any cause, from bereavement to overwork

◆ ME or chronic fatigue syndrome (CFS) (see pages 272–4)

◆ anaemia

◆ poor nutrition

◆ insomnia

◆ illness

◆ fear or phobia due to bad experience or ignorance

◆ being turned off by your partner

◆ childbirth (see page 189).

A common element of many of these factors is an overwhelming loss of energy. If you are not receiving sufficient nourishment, either through illness or poor eating habits, your energy levels will drop dramatically. Lack of sleep or persistent fatigue from being a new parent or a condition such as CFS similarly leave you chronically tired. Worry is a great drain on energy, and a mind constantly preoccupied with annoying thoughts will channel energy into other parts of your life, so sex takes a back seat.

An aversion to sex is slightly different. Early experiences that are confusing or painful can lead to a fear of sexual intercourse. An uncaring or selfish partner (which could mean anything from halitosis to regular premature ejaculation or lack of finesse) can take the pleasure out of sexual encounters, while a traumatic experience such as rape or sexual abuse may require psychiatric help to rediscover an ability to enjoy sex.

## SEXUAL HYSTERIA

In Greek, hysteria means 'twisting of the uterus' and this is the name given to a psychological condition caused primarily by unfulfilled sexual desire.

Girls brought up in cultures in which sex and sexual relationships are a taboo topic sometimes still arrive at their marriage bed uneducated about what to expect. Their first sexual encounters may have been painful but have excited them without bringing them to orgasm. This strange type of fit is a form of outlet that does not occur when they are on their own but exclusively when they have an audience. Even though unconscious, these women can feel pain, and pinching or acupressure on trigger points can bring them back to their senses.

Educating such women and their partners on sexual matters, and encouraging gentleness and care on both sides, usually resolves the problem, which disappears when women begin to enjoy intercourse.

## TOO OLD FOR SEX?

There is absolutely no reason why, as you get older, sex should become a thing of the past, but there are physical reasons why it may lose its appeal. In the wake of the menopause, vaginal dryness, shrinking of nipples and clitoris and less elasticity in the vaginal walls (reducing the dilation and contraction that brings pleasure during intercourse), can make lovemaking much less pleasurable. Lower energy levels and less frequent lovemaking can also lead to less interest in sex. Some women feel under pressure if their partner's libido is as high as ever, for fear of him turning elsewhere. Hormone replacement therapy wards off the effects of the menopause, but you may prefer instead to use natural phyto-oestrogens and supplements. Regular exercise also keeps your energy and stamina levels high and your joints supple, which help retain your enjoyment of lovemaking.

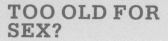

**Treatments**

*Diet:*

◆ Reduce the amount you eat of foods that produce fermentation in the gut, which leads to fatigue: yeast products, excess sugar, blue cheese and canned products.

◆ A high-protein diet maintains optimum blood pressure and helps combat fatigue. A simple protein supplement is 10 almonds soaked in water for 24 hours, then skinned and eaten with a little honey every morning.

◆ Reduce your intake of coffee and alcohol.

## Foods recommended for improving a woman's libido include:

rhubarb
nuts: almonds, pistachios, Brazils, pecans, walnuts, hazelnuts
saffron
yams
ginger
pomegranates
soya
avocado
cherries
apricots
mild green chillies
honey
soft-boiled eggs
spices: asafoetida, coriander, mustard
rhododendron flower chutney
(a traditional Himalayan recipe)

Some of the above may help because of their phyto-oestrogen content.

*Massage:*

The skin is a powerful sensory organ, and it can generate strong emotions when stimulated. Massaging each other can increase mutual attraction and arouse sexual feeling. The style of massage can also vary the effect: pummelling and kneading stimulates the body, while light scratching gently excites, and stroking or touching softly with the fingertips is highly sensuous and relaxing.

*Supplements:*

◆ supplements containing balanced quantities of natural products and phyto-oestrogens help to regulate the hormones.

◆ zinc and magnesium often improve libido.

# Painful coitus

Pain during sexual intercourse is very distressing, and the memory of the pain may persist and interfere with pleasure on subsequent occasions. Vaginismus is the painful reflex spasm of the wall of the vagina, inner muscles of the thighs and the vulva in anticipation of penetration. This can occur in young women who have had no preparation for sex, but trauma rather than ignorance is more likely these days. Gentle care, counselling and patience will be needed to overcome a problem of this sort, with relaxation techniques as part of the therapy.

# Contact bleeding

Bleeding after intercourse should be investigated, in case it is a sign of cervical erosion or ulceration, polyps, cancer or a vaginal infection. Do not delay reporting it to your doctor if you have any problems.

# MASSAGE POINTS

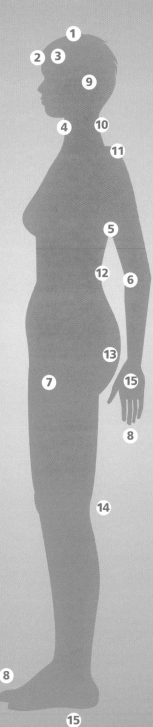

**1 Scalp**
relaxes the body, induces sleep

**2 Forehead**
eases tension and stress

**3 Eyebrows and eyelids**
removes fatigue, eye strain,
creates alertness

**4 Front of neck**
sensitive, causes laughter,
erogenous

**5 Armpit**
ticklish, causes laughter

**6 Inner side of elbows**
erogenous and can help a
paralysed person to enjoy
sexual pleasure

**7 Groin, inner thighs,
pubic region, genitalia**
highly erogenous

**8 Fingers and toes**
pain-relieving and soothing

**9 Back of ears**
erogenous, stimulates body

**10 Back of neck**
removes fatigue, headache,
stress, anxiety, and improves
blood flow to the brain
(including hypothalamus,
assisting sexual function)

**11 Shoulder**
removes fatigue, creates
alertness

**12 Back (entire)**
relaxing, erogenous, removes
fatigue

**13 Sacral area and buttocks**
erogenous

**14 Kneecap and behind
knee**
causes slight agitation

**15 Palms and soles of feet**
relaxing, sensation of being
cared for

# Contraception

Seeking to prevent unwanted pregnancies is nothing new. Herbal brews, magical incantations, lengths of animal guts used as primitive condoms or just trusting to coitus interruptus were all used for centuries.

Perhaps the greatest development in approach to contraception came with the Pill in the 1960s, which, rather than working as a sperm barrier or early abortificant, actually changed a woman's hormonal cycle and prevented ovulation.

Today there is a wide choice of contraceptive methods. The best one for you depends on your individual circumstances – your age and fertility, health history, preference and the importance to you of avoiding pregnancy.

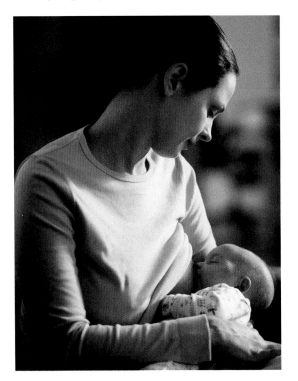

## Coitus interruptus

Withdrawing the penis just before ejaculation places heavy reliance on the man to exert self-control and can be unfulfilling if he reaches the point of orgasm before his partner. It is also not risk-free, as some sperm can precede ejaculation. This is a method that should be avoided unless you feel it wouldn't matter if you became pregnant.

## Breastfeeding

Prolactin, the hormone that triggers milk production, also suppresses ovulation. If you feed your baby exclusively with breast milk you should not ovulate and without ovulation there is no risk of pregnancy. This gift from nature to safeguard against one pregnancy following on too soon after another is theoretically a very effective form of contraception, but has often been misinterpreted. Even a short break in breastfeeding, or supplementing the baby's feeds, reduces the natural protection that prolactin provides, which makes it a particularly risky method of birth control.

# Rhythm method (periodic abstinence)

Simply put, this involves limiting intercourse to when there is no viable egg either in the uterus or Fallopian tubes, so that the sperm can find no egg to fertilize. This can be an effective method of contraception but is dependent on several conditions. Timing is vital, and works as follows:

If you have a 28-day cycle, you are likely to ovulate around the 13th or 14th day of the cycle. The egg is then potent for up to three days (although probably only two). As sperm has a maximum lifespan of five days, intercourse can be safely had up to the eighth day of the cycle followed by a period of abstinence until the 17th day (or use barrier contraception).

It is said that one can get pregnant at any time of the cycle, other than during periods, but such incidences are textbook cases and extremely rare, so in theory the rhythm method is quite safe. However, it does depend on predicting the not-always predictable. Your cycle may be shorter or longer, and circumstances such as stress, travel or illness may alter it. You will have to record your ovulation day over three cycles before you can forecast when you will next ovulate. But what has happened in the past may not hold true in the future, so for extra safety you may want to back up this calendar calculation with mucus and/or temperature readings (specially sensitive thermometers are available) – see Infertility, page 114. You will have to do this anyway if your ovulation day varies, and add days on to the beginning and end of the abstinence period for extra security.

The rhythm method has the advantages of no medical side-effects; it is also the only contraceptive method sanctioned by the Roman Catholic church. Its effectiveness, however, depends on a highly regular cycle and a vigilant eye on the calendar.

| | |
|---|---|
| 1 2 3 4 | period — SAFE PERIOD |
| 5 6 7 8 | SAFE PERIOD |
| 9 10 11 12 13 14 15 16 17 | ovulate — ABSTINENCE |
| 18 19 20 21 22 23 24 25 26 27 28 | SAFE PERIOD |

# Vaginal douches

Using a post-coital douche to flush out the semen is not recommended as a form of pregnancy prevention. Sperm swim very fast and can be found on the cervix of the uterus within 90 seconds of ejaculation, so even proprietary hygiene products with a spermicidal additive are not safe, let alone plain or salt water, vinegar or lemon juice. I once came across a woman who had tried her own version using antiseptic cream, which had given her severe vaginitis.

# Barrier methods

## CONDOM OR SHEATH

Used properly, condoms are an effective and inexpensive form of contraceptive, and also provide protection against the spread of sexually transmitted infections. Many are impregnated with spermicide, and spermicidal cream or jelly increases their safety and reduces the risk of fertilization in the unlikely event that the condom should split. A condom may become damaged if not removed carefully from its packaging, by incorrect application or if the latex rubber has lost strength because it has exceeded its shelf life. Men sometimes complain about a dulled sense of feeling or loss of spontaneity, although the latter can be overcome by incorporating the putting on of the condom into foreplay.

Female condoms are more expensive and bulkier than male condoms, but are also very reliable and give the woman control over contraception.

## DIAPHRAGM OR CAP

Like a condom, a cervical diaphragm or cap provides a barrier that interrupts the sperm's passage towards the egg, but is reusable rather than a one-time, throw-away item. A diaphragm is a flexible rubber dome that fits inside the vagina right across the width and is held in place by a spring. The cap is smaller and more rigid, and is shaped to fit over the cervix at the entrance to the uterus. Both are used with a spermicidal jelly, and can be inserted several hours before intercourse; they must be left in place for several hours afterwards.

Size is important: too tight can cause irritation due to friction; too loose and its effectiveness will be compromised. Your diaphragm should be fitted by a trained healthcare professional who will show you how to insert and remove it, and instruct you in its use and care – scrupulous hygiene is also important.

Correctly inserted and not removed prematurely, diaphragms have a good safety record. Failures usually come from incorrect size or fitting. Rubber does perish, so you should replace your diaphragm about once a year, when you should also be checked to ensure that the fit is still correct – any internal changes may mean a different size is required.

Diaphragms have the advantage over condoms of being in the woman's control and, as long as she has taken the precaution of inserting it beforehand, not interrupting lovemaking in the early stages. Some women get the hang of inserting them more easily than others.

# Intra-uterine device (IUD)

This small device, also called the IUCD (intra-uterine contraceptive device), loop or coil, is made of plastic or metal or both. It is introduced into the uterus through the cervical canal and can remain in place for a year or longer.

Despite different models of IUD having been available for many years, it is still not completely understood how they work. Being a foreign body in the uterus, the IUD affects the quality of the endometrium, the uterus lining, and may also make it physically more difficult for an egg to implant successfully. Copper in an IUD also affects the endometrium as the metal gradually ionizes.

The most common side-effect of an IUD is to make periods heavier and more prolonged, so if your periods are already heavy this may not be the best option. After perhaps a little initial discomfort on fitting (done by a qualified person), you should not otherwise be aware of the device. For some women, however, it can be the cause of continued cramp and discomfort, spotting or bleeding, or vaginal discharge that may indicate pelvic infection. If this happens, your doctor or family planning adviser will usually want to remove the IUD.

A variation on the standard IUD is a coil that contains a synthetic hormone, progestin, which it slowly releases. This causes periods to stop and can provide contraception for up to five years. If it doesn't suit you, side-effects from the progestin may include acne, depression, headaches or hormonal weight gain.

It is occasionally possible for a fertilized egg to develop despite the presence of an IUD. If this happens, the IUD needs to be removed as quickly as possible, but its removal may trigger a spontaneous abortion. There is also a slightly increased risk of ectopic pregnancy (i.e. outside the uterus, see page 147). It is possible for an IUD to be spontaneously expelled, most likely during menstruation, so it is necessary to check that the device is in place (a small cord that extends down into the vagina enables you to do this).

# Hormonal contraception

### THE PILL

The active ingredients in the contraceptive pill are synthetic steroids similar to the natural female sex hormones, in doses designed to inhibit ovulation.

The combination pill – containing oestrogen and progestogen – is typically taken daily for 21 days, followed by a seven-day break, to make up a 28-day cycle. To avoid losing count, packets often contain 28 pills, to be taken in order. The final seven pills are, in effect, placebos, as they don't contain any hormones.

Most complications of the contraceptive pill are due to oestrogen, which led to the development of lower-dose pills (early forms of the pill contained five times or more oestrogen than most current formulas).

The mini-pill or progestogen-only pill avoids oestrogen altogether. Without oestrogen, the mini-pill does not stop ovulation, but triggers the production of thick mucus discharge at the opening of the cervix, which bars sperm from entering the uterus. Should any get through, the progestogen also acts on the endometrium (uterus lining) to prevent an egg from implanting itself.

Without ovulation there is no real menstruation, but the seven-day break triggers 'withdrawal bleeding', which is much the same in practical terms, although often rather lighter. It is possible your periods may stop altogether: some women welcome this, but others prefer the additional reassurance that they are not pregnant.

The pills need to be taken regularly and in the right order (with some systems there may be two or three different formulas within a month's supply). Missing even one or two can negate the contraceptive effect. The lower the dose, the more precision is necessary, and very low-dose combination pills and mini-pills should be taken at the same time every day.

The contraceptive pill, provided it is taken correctly, is reassuringly effective, but not without certain risks.

### Side-effects

Reactions vary, both from individual to individual and from pill to pill. Some women may complain of cyclical headaches or breast tenderness, while others find exactly the same symptoms clear up when they are on the pill. Fluid retention, weight gain and a slight increase in blood pressure are common effects that are not necessarily a problem but should be monitored.

When taken over a long period (five years or more), the pill can sometimes have greater side-effects.

A regular supplement of hormones disturbs your hormonal system. When you stop taking the contraceptive pill, it may take time for your body to re-establish its natural balance and cycle. Fertility may not return for a year or so; there is more work to be done on the difficulty of conceiving after prolonged use of the pill.

The synthetic hormones are metabolized (de-activated or destroyed) by the liver, and taking the pill long-term can impair the liver function. One of the side-effects of this is to affect the liver's ability to control blood clotting, which leads to danger from stroke, pulmonary embolism and deep vein thrombosis.

I have always cautioned young girls about the use of contraceptive pills. Teenage pregnancy is on the rise and has become a major social problem, but if you tamper with nature, then your body is more likely to go wrong. I have known five young women who have suffered a stroke while on the pill.

Another function of the liver is to produce enough bile for the digestive system. Bile is a natural suppressant of yeast and candida growth in the gut. Contraceptive pills are often linked to candida overgrowth, resulting not

## PILL PROBLEMS

If you vomit within a few hours of taking the pill, or have severe diarrhoea, you may not be protected. In that case continue taking the pill but use additional protection, such as a condom, for the next seven days. Some medications, such as antibiotics and complementary medicines, can make the pill less effective. If you are unsure, ask the advice of a doctor or nurse and use additional protection such as condoms. If you forget to take a contraceptive pill, the steps you should take will mainly depend on the type of pill you are using.

### COMBINED PILL

◆ **Less than 12 hours late taking the pill:** take the last pill you missed and continue with the rest of the pills as normal. If there are less than 7 pills left after the missed pill, continue with the pack and go on to the next pack the following day: don't leave the usual 7-day break.

◆ **More than 12 hours late taking the pill:** take the last pill you missed and use a condom for the next seven days. Do not leave the usual 7-day break.

### EVERY DAY COMBINED PILL

◆ **More than 12 hours late taking the pill:** take the last pill you missed and use a condom for the next seven days. If there are less than seven active pills left in the pack, take those as normal, and then continue with the next active pill, missing out on the larger inactive pills.

### PROGESTOGEN-ONLY PILL

◆ **Less than three hours late taking the pill:** take it as soon as you remember and the next one at the usual time.

◆ **More than three hours late taking the pill:** take it as soon as you remember and the next one at the usual time (even if this means taking two at once). If you have forgotten more than one pill, take the last one you missed and the next one at the usual time and use a condom for the next two days.

## IN ADDITION TO CONTRACEPTION

The right type of pill for you can have positive side-effects, and may prove beneficial to problems such as:

- menstrual cramps
- PMS
- breast tenderness
- very heavy periods
- unpredictable periods
- anaemia from irregular or excessive bleeding
- polycystic ovaries
- hirsutism
- acne
- abdominal pains associated with endometriosis (see pages 104–6)

only in digestive problems, but fungal outbreaks in other areas, such as thrush and athlete's foot.

Increasing the oestrogen in the body over time may also increase the risk of breast cancer (see page 202). The mini-pill slightly increases the risk of ectopic pregnancy.

### MORNING-AFTER PILL (POST-COITAL EMERGENCY CONTRACEPTION)

The most common form of treatment involves giving high-dose tablets of an oestrogen derivative within 72 hours of intercourse. If taken on time, the effectiveness is about 75 per cent. The most common side-effects are nausea and sickness, headaches, fatigue and a general feeling of being unwell for a few days.

The progestogen-only post-coital pill is better tolerated. The sudden surge of hormones in the blood confuses the body and the endometrium becomes non-receptive to a fertilized egg. These hormones give a false message to the pituitary, which temporarily stops producing luteinizing hormone.

### HORMONAL CONTRACEPTION BY INJECTION OR IMPLANTATION

An increasingly popular alternative to taking hormones orally every day is to have a periodic injection or implant. Depending on the strength and combination of hormones used, these can provide protection for up to a year. The hormones interfere with the pituitary's mid-cycle production of luteinizing hormone and ovulation is suppressed. The imbalance caused by this suppression means the endometrium may not develop so well, resulting in menstruation that is either irregular or suppressed.

Menstruation may continue to be absent for a year or so after this form of contraception ceases. Other possible side-effects may include: headaches, fatigue, dizziness, nervousness and abdominal discomfort from pain or bloating. The low oestrogen levels in the blood may reduce bone density (see Osteoporosis, page 308).

## Sterilization

Sealing or severing the Fallopian tubes cuts off the egg's route to the uterus. Although in theory the operation can be reversed, the success rate is not good and this should be considered a permanent form of contraception. For this reason you will be asked many questions about your circumstances and reasons for wanting sterilization, and you should carefully consider all the pros and cons before proceeding. The operation is usually done under general anaesthetic, using keyhole surgery, so recovery is quicker than it would be with open surgery, although you will still need to take things easy for a week or two.

If you are in a steady relationship the question of which of you should be operated upon will arise. A vasectomy for a man is a less involved operation, but this needs to be weighed against your own particular feelings and requirements, and also what may happen in the future.

# Sexually Transmitted Infections (STIs) As recently as 20 years ago, STIs were usually lumped together under the umbrella 'VD', or venereal disease.

Vital though it is to curb the spread of HIV and AIDS, it is the more common infections that are worrying – precisely because they are so widespread. It is estimated that up to 1 in 20 women under the age of 30 have chlamydia and up to 30 per cent have had it in the past.

Women are more vulnerable to STIs than men. They don't get infected more frequently, but they are more likely to be asymptomatic – where a man may be warned by a sore or lesion on his penis, a woman may be quite unaware of a similar sore on her cervix and so not seek treatment at an early stage. Also, when untreated infection spreads internally, it can cause damage to the reproductive system, leading to sterility.

Despite the blanket label, not all STIs are only transmitted by sexual contact. Personal hygiene plays a part in the transmission of some infections, and some can be passed from mother to child, either while still in the womb or during birth.

## HIV AND PREGNANCY

If an HIV+ woman becomes pregnant she stands a better than even chance of passing the virus on to her baby before it is born. A decision to have an abortion is never easy, even in such circumstances, so it is important to get impartial expert advice on the best way to proceed, and to discuss things with your partner. If you come to the conclusion that abortion is not an option, seek out sympathetic support. You will be offered antiviral drugs (such as AZT), which reduce the risk of your baby acquiring the virus.

## HELPING YOURSELF AND OTHERS

Most STIs can be effectively and simply treated. The problem is realizing there is a problem if there are no early symptoms. This leads to the single biggest concern: the ease with which STIs can be passed on and proliferate.

The more widespread an infection or disease is, the greater the likelihood of catching it. So, in the realm of public health, the aim of doctors, genito-urinary clinics and so on is not just early diagnosis and effective treatment of individual patients, but curtailing the spread. Until reliable vaccines are found that work in all cases, the best methods are education and protection. On a personal level, this means:

- being informed of the different types of STI. Statistically, your chances of becoming HIV+ are very low, but the chances of being infected by genital warts or chlamydia are very high, and both of these can threaten your overall health if not treated.

- not exposing yourself to unprotected sex with a partner of whom you are not sure.

- going for a check-up if you have any concerns, even if you have no symptoms.

- following any treatment fully.

- being honest and open about sexual contacts when asked. (Clinical staff have heard it all before, so don't allow embarrassment to stand in the way of efforts to limit infection in others.)

# Chlamydia

Chlamydial infections are on the rise, and infection by Chlamydia trachomatis is the most common form of STI in girls and women. Because chlamydia is widespread, the chance of recurrence from contact with different sexual partners is also a constant worry, leading to suspicion and tension in a relationship.

A smelly vaginal discharge with inflammation of the cervix may warn of infection, but more often there are no symptoms. Undetected, chlamydia can lead to tubal blockages and pelvic inflammatory disease, with subsequent infertility. It can also cause complications in pregnancy, increase the likelihood of ectopic pregnancy (see page 147), bring on premature labour and spread infection in the Fallopian tubes after delivery. The infection can be passed on from a mother to her newborn baby.

Although not a life-threatening disease, chlamydia can have disproportionate consequences many years after infection. To discover at 30 that you cannot have children, because of an infection you never knew you had a decade or more earlier, can be devastating.

Diagnosis is by a simple laboratory test. It may be discovered as a result of a precautionary check-up or on a routine gynaecological examination. Sexually active women under 20 years of age are two to three times more likely to have chlamydia than others, so screening sexually active teenagers is a sensible measure.

Treatment is a straightforward course of antibiotics. All women treated for chlamydia should subsequently be screened every three to four months.

# Herpes simplex

The virus Herpesvirus hominis is the most common cause of genital ulcers, or herpes. It is referred to as HSV2 to differentiate it from HSV1 (herpes or cold sores around the mouth or nostrils), but the two cross-infect, so someone with a cold sore on their lip, for example, could infect you with genital herpes in the course of oral sex.

After an incubation period of two to seven days, small blisters appear on the labia and inside the vagina, often heralded by tingling, burning and itching. When these eruptions burst they form small, painful ulcers. There may be a watery discharge, urination may be frequent or difficult, and often people feel tired and feverish. Sexual intercourse is painful, but you should abstain anyway, because the infectious period lasts for as long as there are visible signs and for up to a week afterwards.

These ulcers may persist for two to six weeks and then heal without scars. The ulcers heal on their own, indicating the body has developed some sort of immunity. Recurrent attacks can be expected, but with fewer, smaller ulcers that heal more quickly.

The virus travels not in the blood but through the nervous system, which accounts for the burning or tingling sensations in affected nerve endings. Although you are not infectious between attacks, the virus does not disappear, but goes dormant, retreating to the ganglion of nerves near the spine.

Since the ulcers heal themselves, treatment is mostly a matter of relieving the symptoms. Loose-fitting cotton underwear, careful genital hygiene and cool compresses all help minimize aggravation, and painkillers are helpful. I often recommend neem (margosa) oil, which has some antiviral properties, or marigold oil or cream (as used for verrucas), which may give quicker relief.

Women who suffer from regular recurrences (perhaps as often as once a month) are often helped by a prescription of acyclovir, an antiviral drug. It is often said that frequent intercourse may cause recurrent herpes, but flare-ups are more likely when you are run down or stressed. Following the Lifestyle Programme has for many women reduced the frequency of their attacks.

# Genital warts

These warts may appear on the labia, within the vagina or on the cervix and, though small, cluster together to resemble miniature cauliflowers. They are caused by papilloma viruses and are related to warts you might get on your fingers and elsewhere. However, unlike herpes, you cannot catch genital warts from other forms of warts.

Genital warts are contagious and you should refrain from sexual intercourse until treatment has been completed. During pregnancy, they tend to grow rapidly and should be treated before delivery, as they can be passed from mother to baby during birth.

They may also sometimes be an indicator of pre-cancerous cells on the cervix, so a diagnosis will usually be followed up by a check-up and biopsy.

Standard treatment is to paint the warts with dienlorocetic acid once a week until they disappear (this can take several weeks). They can also be treated with lasers or cryosurgery (using liquid nitrogen to freeze the warts). Herbal remedies such as thuja, marigold product and neem (margosa) oil can be helpful.

# Gonorrhoea

The bacterium *Neisseria gonorrhoea* thrives mainly in the urethra but can be found in the cervix, anal canal and throat. There is a short incubation period of three to five days. The infection is initially asymptomatic, but later symptoms include a thick, greyish, often smelly vaginal discharge, frequent urination, rectal discomfort and itching or burning in the vulva, vagina, cervix and urethra, where the bacteria thrive.

If not treated, the infection can spread, causing skin rashes, swelling in joints and in the tendons of the hands and feet, meningitis and endocarditis (inflammation of the inner lining of the heart). Infection in the Fallopian tubes can cause scarring and, later, infertility. Pelvic inflammation may follow. Babies born to mothers with gonorrhoea may be blinded by the infection.

Gonorrhoea needs to be treated with antibiotics. The disease often goes hand in hand with other sexually transmitted infections, which should be identified and treated at the same time. Sexual partners must also receive treatment; there will need to be a cessation in sexual intercourse until after the treatment is complete.

# Syphilis

Syphilis is once again on the rise. It is only passed between adults by direct sexual contact with an infected partner, but an infected pregnant woman can pass the disease on to her unborn baby.

The first sign of infection shows within 90 days, but usually in about 20 to 30 days. It appears as a sore, known as a *chancre*, on the site of infection, which may be on the lips or nipples as well as in or around the vagina or anus. This sore is not painful and may heal spontaneously within a month or so. The lymph nodes in the groin may also become enlarged but, again, not painful. A danger with syphilis is that, if the *chancre* is deep inside the vagina or on the cervix, it may come and go undetected.

If there are any doubts in the wake of a sexual encounter, it is essential to be checked. Blood tests will be done every six weeks or so, until a positive result is seen. At this stage it is called primary syphilis, and is cured with a complete course of antibiotics that will kill off the infectious organism, *Treponema pallidum*.

If not stopped in this primary stage, syphilis develops into its secondary form, spread via the bloodstream all over the body. There may be fever, swelling of lymph nodes and, distinctively, a skin rash across the torso or palms and soles that doesn't disappear for weeks. There could be patchy alopecia on the scalp, hepatitis and kidney infections.

Left untreated, syphilis will pass into its tertiary phase after years of apparent dormancy. It can act on the central nervous system, causing any number of terrible symptoms. This final phase, less common now thanks to earlier and more successful treatment, was often called GPI, 'general paralysis of the insane'.

# HIV and AIDS

Unlike gonorrhoea, which has been around for millennia, HIV (human immunodeficiency virus) is a mutated retrovirus that has been a threat for only around 30 years. The virus thrives in the T lymphocytes, the white blood cells responsible for immune responses. Normally, these lymphocytes destroy invading bacteria and viruses, and develop antibodies to combat further attacks. When this defence system fails to work properly, invading cells can't be destroyed nor antibodies developed. As a result, opportunistic infections are a constant danger.

## HOW THE VIRUS DEVELOPS

If you are HIV+ (diagnosed by a blood test), your weakened immune system leaves you in danger of developing AIDS (acquired immune deficiency syndrome). The usual progression, often after many years without apparent symptoms, is to develop a chronic fever and fatigue, with swollen glands, diarrhoea and loss of weight. This is not AIDS but described as AIDS-related complex (ARC). For some, this is a precursor to full-blown AIDS, but others recover, not ridding themselves of the virus but not succumbing to AIDS either.

Without an effective immune system, the body is defenceless and subject to one disease after another. Kaposi's sarcoma is a particular form of tumour associated with AIDS, often seen as a bluish-black lump occurring on the skin or other organs. Meningitis, blindness and dementia are not uncommon.

## THE RISKS

The virus travels from person to person via bodily fluids, predominantly semen or vaginal secretions and blood, although it is present in breast milk, saliva, urine and excreta. Contact needs to be direct, which is why the most usual ways of contracting HIV are unprotected sex, contaminated needles or a baby from its mother.

Stringent precautions are taken with blood for transfusions and all medical procedures, but risks from these sources exist in some parts of the world. Normal social contact does not spread the virus, and health workers do not catch it from patients. It cannot penetrate unbroken skin or lie in wait on toilet seats.

With no cure yet available, avoidance is paramount. The precautions against STIs outlined on page 138 apply particularly to HIV because of the long period when a carrier is infectious but has no symptoms. A strong person with a previously healthy immune system can bear the virus with little effects for many years, but could pass it on to others for whom it is an early death knell.

## TREATMENTS

Individual infections can be treated according to their nature (Kaposi's sarcoma by surgery or radiotherapy, pneumonia with long-term antibiotics, and so on), and there are expensive drugs available that aim to bolster up a failing immune system, but nothing has yet been found that actually kills the virus.

What is recognized to make a big difference is a two-pronged approach to support your weakened immune system: living as healthy a lifestyle as possible and shielding your body as far as possible from infection.

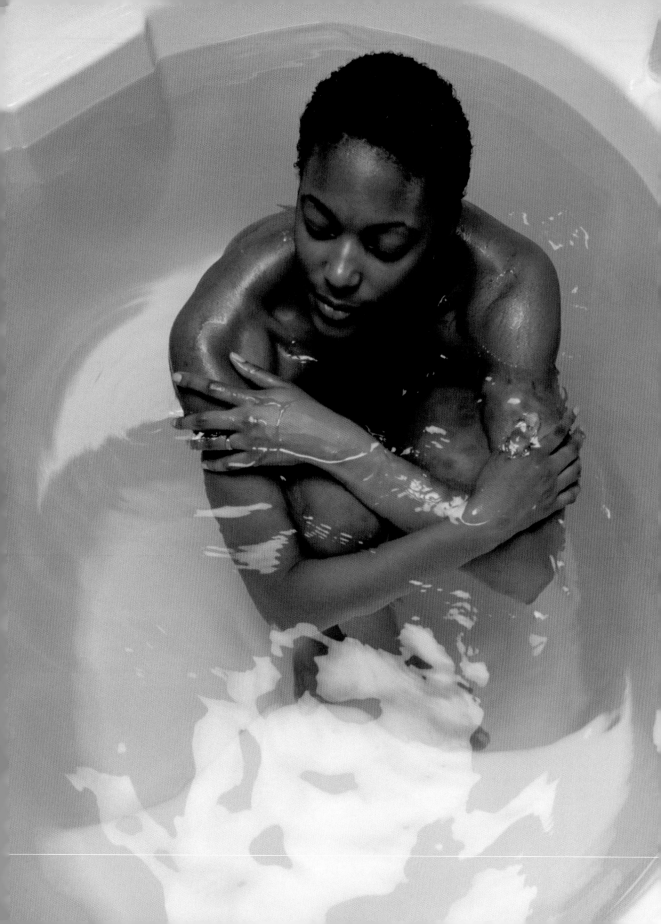

## HYGIENE ...

With this disease, the very backbone of the immune system is broken down. Instead of strengthening your body's ability to combat infection, every exposure weakens it further, so it is vital to protect yourself against minor infections that a healthy immune system would shrug off without difficulty. Cuts and scrapes, dirt from everyday life, the common cold, will all have a debilitating effect.

Avoid exposing yourself to others' ailments. Friends will understand that they should not visit you when they are feeling under the weather. You may need to find an alternative, for instance, to travelling on crowded public transport (where not only coughs and colds circulate freely, but serious diseases such as TB are becoming a major worry in some cities). Wearing a mask will help shield you from inhaling airborne germs.

Scrupulous cleanliness will help prevent infection reaching your body. This ranges from washing your hands before and after every activity to keeping your home hygienic and dirt-free.

All bodily orifices and crevices are potential entry points for infection:

■ Bathe at least once a day, and be scrupulous about washing every part of your body, especially your genitalia, between your toes and your navel. Wet wipes are a useful standby.

■ As well as cleaning your teeth and gums, floss and gargle with a weakened solution of potassium permanganate (what dentists use as a rinse). See personal hygiene (page 293) for maintaining gum health.

## A DAILY NASAL DOUCHE

Stir and dissolve ⅔ teaspoon of table salt into a 250ml tumbler of lukewarm water. Pour some on to your palms and suck into your nostrils, or use a nose dropper. Alternatively, if you can find an Indian inhaler known as a jal neti (netipot), you could use this to inhale the saline solution.

■ Splash your eyes with cold water two or three times a day, and gently remove any accumulations in the corners of your eyes, especially when you wake up.

■ Once a week, pour a drop of organic olive oil or pure mustard or mullein oil (available from homeopathic shops) into each ear at bedtime to soften accumulated wax so that it can be gently removed.

● Keep your nails short.

● Blow your nose several times a day, even if it feels clean. Mucus is an ideal nutrient for bacteria.

## ... AND HEALTH

The ideal would be to move to a mountain retreat, a sanctuary where the air is pure and you can be as close to nature as possible, to eat only organic food and follow a regime of light exercise, rest and meditation.

For most people this is not a realistic move, but it is necessary to treat both your body and mind as well as possible to maintain optimum energy and well-being. See the chapter on General Disorders and Problems for care in long-term or terminal illness.

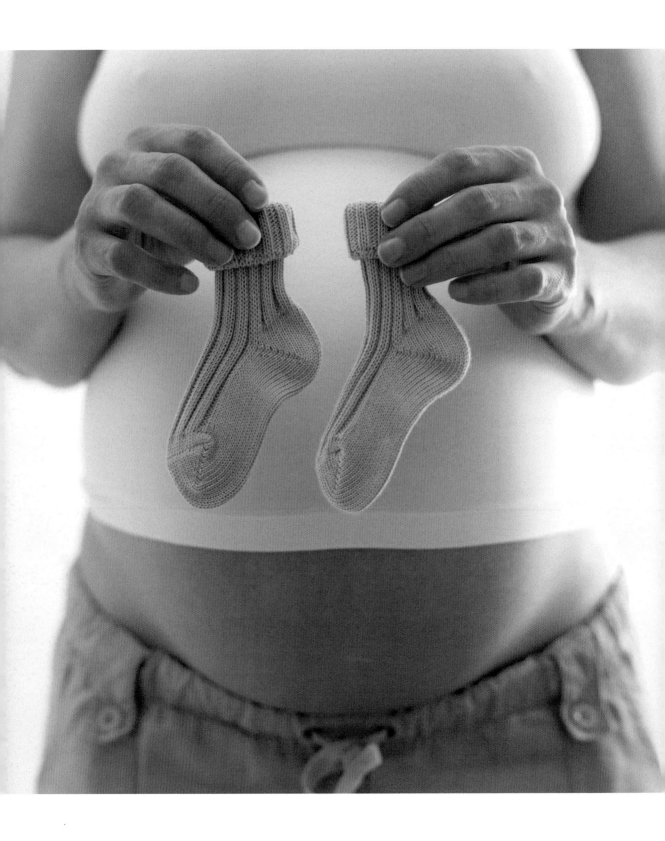

# chapter three

# pregnancy

Bearing a child is one of the most natural things in the world, but the process can be a mixed blessing: fearful as well as exciting, tiring as well as rewarding. As medical knowledge has grown, so has intervention in all stages of pregnancy and birth. This means that far fewer women and babies die in childbirth, complications can be dealt with early, before they become serious, and newborn babies who are premature or sick have a much higher chance of survival. However, it also means that pregnancy has sometimes come to be seen as a medical 'condition' that needs 'treating', and women feel further removed and less in control of the whole business.

# The most natural thing in the world?

## It is, but pregnancy can seem to many women like a scary, complicated process.

On one of my training programmes, NHS doctors visited a local primary care centre in a remote part of Rajasthan. They saw women coming in after their waters had broken and being helped by the midwife at the final stages of labour as they squatted on the floor (the most natural position) and gave birth. The women then rested for a couple of hours and went home on bullock carts. These doctors were amazed how quick the entire thing was. Most women in regions like this deliver at home and hardly ever come into contact with medicine, and the population is growing healthily. Why are things so much more complicated and harassed here in the West?

In traditional societies, women know about every stage of pregnancy and it is a knowledge that is passed on from generation to generation. In the more developed parts of the world, grandmothers, mothers and mothers-in-law now no longer pass on tried and tested values on nutrition, hygiene, rest, peace, exercise and habits during pregnancy, and women turn to books and the medical establishment for advice.

## Planning for pregnancy

Your experience of pregnancy has much to do with how well your body is prepared for it beforehand. Many of the uncomfortable symptoms of pregnancy and some of the more serious complications that sometimes arise can be averted or alleviated if you are healthy and well nourished, your muscles toned and you are practised in relaxation techniques. The Lifestyle Programme is a good guide to preparing your body for pregnancy.

## RISK FACTORS

For some women, becoming pregnant carries a higher risk than usual. Before you move ahead with your plans for having a child, you should talk to your doctor and consider the implications if you are affected by any of the risk factors listed below. Some pose a more serious health danger than others, but in all cases it is important that you and your doctor are alerted so that appropriate precautions can be taken.

Serious risks to pregnancy are posed by a history of:

◆ miscarriage or habitual abortion (three or more)
◆ pre-term deliveries or stillbirths
◆ pre-eclampsia
◆ infections such as tuberculosis, AIDS or sexually transmitted diseases.

If you have already had a child with a genetic or congenital disorder, you will want to discuss with your doctor implications for subsequent children.

The following also need be taken into consideration:

◆ below the age of 15 or above 40 (extremes of age increase the risk, especially for a first pregnancy)
◆ high blood pressure or history of deep vein thrombosis or blood clots
◆ kidney or heart disease
◆ diabetes
◆ blood incompatibility (Rhesus negative blood type, when your partner is Rhesus positive)
◆ cancer in remission

- obesity
- severe thyroid disorder
- epilepsy
- chronic anaemia
- physical anomalies (such as a small uterus or pelvic deformity)
- surgery or previous infection in your Fallopian tubes
- use of steroids or high doses of immuno-suppressants for diseases like rheumatoid arthritis
- drug abuse
- psychiatric illness (such as manic depression, mental retardation and schizophrenia).

Frequent monitoring by a doctor becomes very important in these situations. An obstetrician is trained to monitor pregnancy and participate in delivery and, for some of the complications mentioned above, will need to call on the expertise of other specialists.

## Confirming pregnancy

A particular hormone in the placenta (HCG) can be detected as early as nine days after fertilization. Pregnancy home-testing kits are designed to detect traces of this hormone in the urine, and if instructions are followed carefully these are quite reliable. An ultrasound examination and a blood test are usually used to confirm pregnancy. Once your pregnancy is confirmed, you will be able to calculate approximately when the baby will be due (see box opposite).

## ESTIMATED DATE OF CONFINEMENT (EDC)

Take the date of your last period, add seven days and then minus three months.

e.g.: if your last period began on 31 March:

31 + 7 = 7 April

April minus 3 months = January

so EDC = 7 January

This is based on a menstrual cycle of 28 days. If your cycle is shorter or longer than this, then adjust the days you add at the beginning accordingly (e.g.: add 5 days if your cycle is 26 days long, or 9 days if it is 30 days long).

### ECTOPIC PREGNANCY

It is customary to have an early scan to ensure that the pregnancy is in the uterus. In a small minority of cases a fertilized egg implants itself somewhere other than in the lining of the womb. In almost all cases this means the Fallopian tubes. This can be very risky especially when undetected (accounting for about 10 per cent of maternal deaths in pregnancy). The chance of an ectopic pregnancy increases if you have had an infection in or surgery on your Fallopian tubes – to reverse a sterilization procedure (tubal ligation) or to dilate a tube, for example.

Since periodic spotting may continue during an ectopic pregnancy there may be no early sign until a warning pain is felt, usually on the side where the tubal pregnancy has taken place; you may also experience dizziness, light-headedness or fainting. If the tube ruptures, abdominal pain and haemorrhage become severe and emergency surgery is required. As soon as you suspect something is wrong consult your physician or gynaecologist.

# Physical changes

The stages of pregnancy are generally divided into three three-month periods known as trimesters, although the divisions are only nominal and not precise. By the end of the nine months' gestation a typical uterus will grow from about 8cm in length and 30–40g in weight to 30cm in length and 1.1kg in weight. In addition to the baby itself it will contain the placenta and about 5 litres of amniotic fluid, protecting the growing baby from shocks and allowing it to move and exercise itself.

But your swelling abdomen is only one of the incredible changes that your body undergoes. Your whole body responds to the pregnancy. Some changes happen straight away, others only in the later stages.

■ Most noticeable right from the start is that your heartbeat quickens as it has to circulate a greater volume of blood, which increases by between 40 and 100 per cent, depending on your build. This increase is in response to the requirements of the growing baby and the extra demands of your own body; it will also compensate for some loss of blood at the time of birth.

■ Your breathing rate per minute increases as your oxygen consumption rises by up to 20 per cent, supplying your unborn baby with necessary oxygen. In the later stages you will feel breathless as the baby takes up more and more room.

■ Quite early in pregnancy, your breasts become larger and heavier, and you will probably notice bluish veins. From the second trimester you may start to secrete colostrum, a sort of precursor to proper milk.

■ You will probably find you need to urinate more frequently from quite early on, before you are aware of the growing baby.

■ Relaxation of your digestive tract increases the chances of upsets from heartburn to constipation, especially during the second half of your pregnancy.

■ Other muscles and ligaments also relax and stretch in the later part of pregnancy, which can contribute to backache and flat feet. Even your gums soften.

■ Under hormonal influences your skin and hair will undergo changes. You may go through a 'teenage' stage early on, with greasy hair and even spots, but this is overturned during the second trimester, when many women find their hair grows extra luxuriously and their skin glows – the 'bloom' of pregnancy. You may also find a darker line, the linea negra, appearing down the middle of your abdomen, and some women find pigmentation marks appearing on their face (see Chloasma, page 164).

Although all these changes are expected and natural, they are not all comfortable. However, for most, there are steps you can take to alleviate the symptoms (see Common Complaints, pages 160–4).

## ANTENATAL CLASSES

Antenatal classes are helpful in several ways:
● This is where you can learn and practise exercises that will help ease labour.
● You can learn more about the changes your body is going through, what to expect and what to look out for. Fear of the unknown adds enormously to a mother-to-be's anxiety and increases the pain of childbirth.
● You can share experiences and learn from other pregnant women.

# HORMONAL TRIGGERS

On becoming pregnant, your whole hormonal balance changes; here are just a few triggers for which you will notice the effects:

- Prolactin suppresses ovulation, bringing a halt to the usual menstrual cycle.
- The same hormone triggers the development of breast tissue in preparation for breastfeeding.
- Progesterone secretions ensure the continued growth of the lining of the uterus. Soon the placenta develops and begins to secrete its own hormones, as part of its job is to guarantee a continuous supply of blood and nutrients to the growing baby. Your growth and other hormones govern the baby's development until its own pituitary and thyroid develop.
- At the time of labour the hypothalamus produces oxytocin, which triggers contractions.

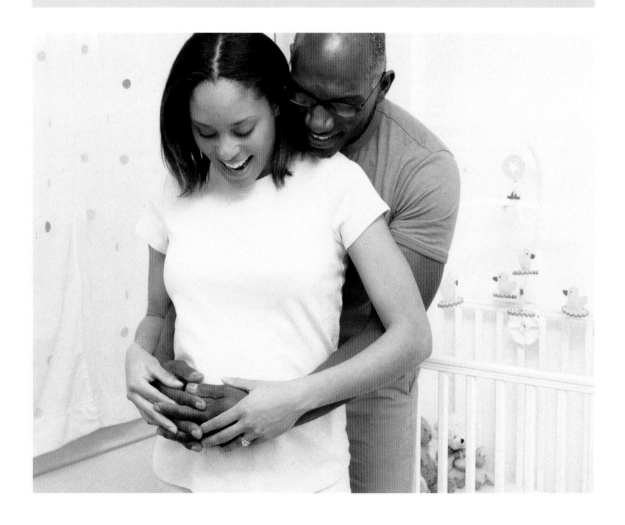

# Keeping yourself healthy

The greater care you take over your health during this time, the better you will feel. Pregnancy will take less of a toll on your body and your innate well-being will make it easier to cope with the quite dramatic upheavals your body is undergoing. You are less likely to need interventions such as drugs and there are likely to be fewer risks to both you and your unborn baby.

Imagine a foetus growing up under extremely stressful conditions, where the mother did not bother and did everything wrong (eating junk food, drinking alcohol, taking drugs and partying), and the baby was then subjected to a traumatic birth with bright hospital lights, shouting and emergency procedures. A frightening start in the world. Why put the baby through so much? Follow a few simple rules and give your child a good start in life.

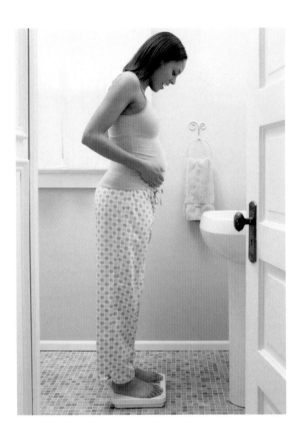

## NUTRITION AND WEIGHT GAIN

The average weight gain during pregnancy is 12.5kg, of which a full-term baby will account for about 3kg. The growth of the placenta, the amniotic fluid, distribution of new fat, growth of breasts and fluid retention make up the rest.

It is easy to think, especially if you are naturally slim, that if you're losing your figure you may as well make the most of it and eat as much as you like of whatever you like. Don't! Although an increase in weight is vital to your health and your growing baby's, it does put a strain on your heart and muscles, so it is important not to add further unnecessary weight by losing control of your intake of sugars and fatty foods.

Although not an ideal way of accounting for what you eat, a calorie count gives a good idea in this instance of how little extra you need. The recommended calorie intake for an average woman is 2,000–2,500 calories,

and this should increase by about 200–350 calories a day during pregnancy – so about 10 per cent more. Because your demand for vitamins and minerals goes up (see box opposite), you may need supplements during pregnancy and breastfeeding.

You should also keep up your water intake of 1½–2 litres a day, even though you may be tempted to restrict your fluids, because of sore breasts, less bladder control and a general puffiness.

In late pregnancy a simple diet is best: fruits, poultry, fish, nuts (soaked), milk, rice, lentils, vegetables and some butter. I recommend fruits that are softer (ripe bananas, plums, nectarines, berries, mangoes, etc.) and soft vegetables, such as spinach, swede, pumpkins, tomatoes, potatoes and okra.

Salt should be restricted during pregnancy but not totally avoided.

# NUTRITIONAL REQUIREMENTS

Following the Lifestyle Programme guidelines will give you a healthy diet to follow all through pregnancy, but you should check in particular that you are getting sufficient of the following:

| | ROLE | RECOMMENDED DAILY AMOUNT | USEFUL SOURCES |
|---|---|---|---|
| PROTEIN | essential for embryonic growth | 50g in second half of pregnancy | 1 steak or 2 eggs, a large salmon steak. Strict vegetarians need to ensure sufficient through cottage cheese, tofu, fungus-based meat substitutes, lentils and pulses; and may need protein supplements |
| CALCIUM | an unborn baby demands calcium for its growing bones, and will if necessary 'steal' it from its mother | 1.5g | dairy produce, broccoli, fish, meat, asparagus |
| IRON | vital to blood production; too little causes anaemia | 50mg | meat, fish, eggs, leafy vegetables, dried fruit; see also Liver, page 166 |
| VITAMIN C | for bone, skin and cartilage development; aids iron absorption | 500mg | leafy vegetables, sweet peppers, blackcurrants, sweeter varieties of clementine/satsuma |
| FOLATE (FOLIC ACID) | foetal development (preventing spina bifida) | 400mg | pulses, fortified breads and breakfast cereals; supplements usually recommended as diet unlikely to yield sufficient for a pregnant woman |
| ZINC | general growth and development of immune system | 15mg | lean meat, wholegrain cereals, nuts and seeds |
| MAGNESIUM | bones and nerves, and use of muscles | 150mg | pulses, nuts, wholegrain cereals |

## PREGNANCY YOGA

*Check all these exercises with your midwife or obstetrician before embarking on a yoga programme.*

### COMPLETE BREATH

This technique helps to increase your lung capacity, to relieve tension in your upper spine and to open out the mid-chest, decongesting the area.

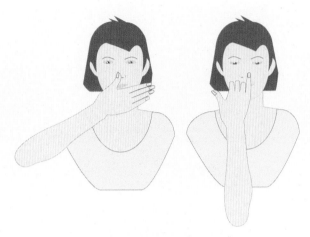

1 Stand or sit cross-legged on the floor. First, breathe out completely. When you inhale, relax your diaphragm by letting go of the area below the ribcage and fill up your lungs slowly and steadily by expanding your chest up and out. Visualize every part of your lungs filling up with air.

2 Now exhale slowly. Try to make your out-breath longer than your in-breath, but stay comfortable. Don't pull in your abdomen – let it relax by itself, so that your lungs remain passive as they empty. Continue for 10 minutes, maintaining the same position and rhythm of breath throughout.

3 When you can perform Steps 1 and 2 without strain, try to hold your breath to achieve a ratio between inhalation, holding and exhalation of 1:1:2. Repeat 20 such breaths. Lie down and relax in the Corpse pose (see page 157).

### ALTERNATIVE NOSTRIL BREATHING

This exercise helps you to control the heating and cooling mechanisms in your body. Breathing through the right nostril creates heat, vitality and alertness, while breathing through the left one has a cooling effect. The pituitary gland in the brain controls this natural thermostat within your body, although its functioning can be disrupted through an insufficient blood supply. This breathing technique allows you to regulate your thermostat more consciously.

1 Sit cross-legged if possible or on a straight-backed chair. Tuck the index and middle fingers of your right hand into your palm or simply use your thumb and index finger. Place your thumb on your right nostril to close it and breathe in deeply through your left nostril.

2 Close your left nostril with your finger and release your thumb. Breathe out completely through your right nostril. Feel your chest muscles relaxing and your shoulders dropping away from your neck as you exhale. Then breathe in through your right nostril.

3 Close your right nostril, release your finger and breathe out through the left one. You have now completed 1 cycle. Continue for 3–5 minutes.

4 Lie down on your back and relax in the Corpse pose (see page 157).

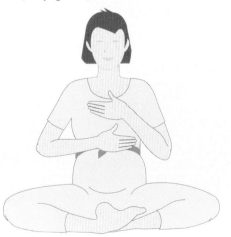

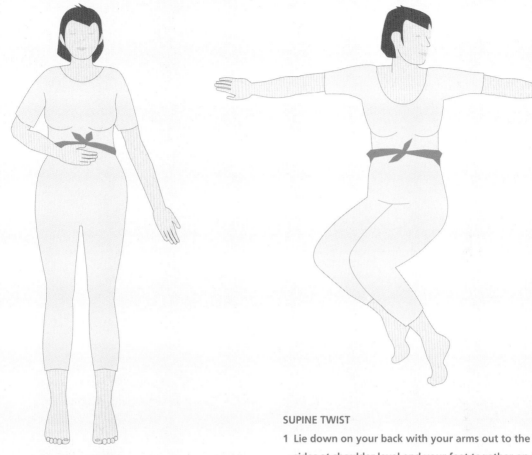

**ABDOMINAL BREATHING**

By moving the diaphragm, this exercise gently massages your internal organs and relaxes the lower abdominal area, thereby improving the blood flow through all the muscles and nerve centres

1 Lie on your back and relax your arms, legs, head and neck completely. Breathe in through your nose and extend your stomach completely, like a balloon filled with air. Avoid arching your back.
2 Breathe out slowly and let your stomach relax. Do not try to pull your stomach muscles in at this stage. Repeat for at least 20 breaths.

**SUPINE TWIST**

1 Lie down on your back with your arms out to the sides at shoulder level and your feet together on the floor, your knees bent.
2 Breathe in, then breathe out and pull in your stomach strongly towards your spine. Lift your knees up to your chest and then lower them towards the floor on the right, at a right angle to your torso. Hold the position and breathe rhythmically, relaxing your upper body completely. Stay for 2–3 breaths, working up to 12 breaths. Then bring your knees up to your chest once more and lower them to the left.
3 Finish by bringing your knees to your chest. Having freed up the chest and main joints, stand up and sit cross-legged to do a few short cleansing breaths.

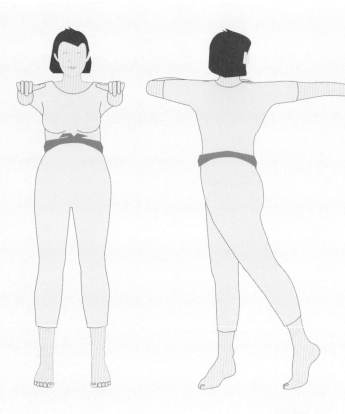

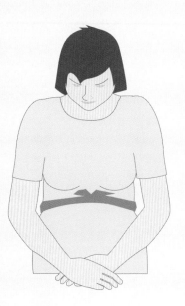

## SWINGING

This will help to improve your vision and relieve fatigue.

1 Stand with your feet about 30 cm apart. Raise your arms up in front of you at shoulder level.

2 Swing to the right by lifting your left heel a little off the floor until your shoulders are in line behind you. Keep your right arm straight while you bend your left arm. Now reverse and swing to the left. Continue swinging from one side to the other, paying attention to moving your head and eyes with your shoulders. As you swing, try not to focus your eyes on any of the objects that appear to be moving rapidly in front of you. Repeat 50 times before going to bed and on waking up in the morning.

## NECK ROLLS

Neck exercises are always useful at night-time for a refreshing sleep.

1 Sit comfortably on a chair, on your heels or cross-legged on the floor. Lower your chin and slowly rotate your neck, first to the right and then to the left, breathing deeply.

2 Finish by inhaling and lowering your chin to your sternum; hold your breath for at least 10 seconds. Release slowly on exhaling, releasing the shoulders.

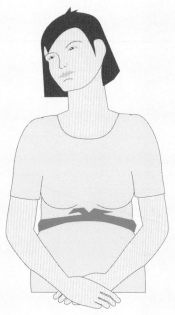

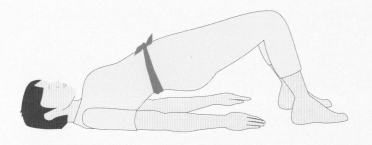

## THE BRIDGE

1 Lie on your back with your arms by your sides, your knees bent and your ankles below your knees, hip-distance apart. Breathe in and peel your back off the floor until just your head, shoulders and feet are in contact with the floor. Keep stretching your neck while your back is lifted. Come down slowly on breathing out. Relax. Repeat 5 times.

2 Repeat Step 1 but this time raise your arms up over your head, stretching your arms away from your shoulders.

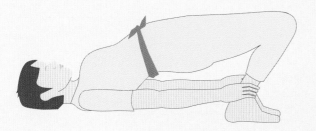

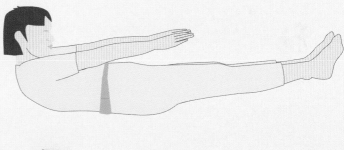

## BOAT POSE

1 Lie on your back with your legs stretched out, feet together, and your hands by the sides of your hips. Take a deep breath in and raise your head, legs and arms off the floor. Breathe out and lower your body to the floor, keeping your eyes level with your feet throughout. Rest. Repeat 5 times.

2 Once you are strong enough, try the full posture shown here. Keep your eyes level with your feet.

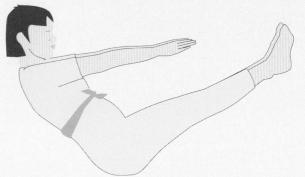

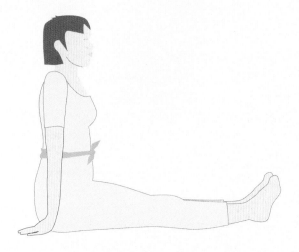

## STICK POSE

1 Sit with your legs extended in front of you and your spine at a right angle to your legs. Place your palms on the floor behind you and open out the front of your shoulders as shown. Lift your spine up to lengthen it, and straighten your neck. Spread out your toes without stretching the back of your heels.

2 Now turn your palms towards your knees, keeping your shoulders turned out. Push your hands down towards the floor for 5 seconds, building up over time to 20 seconds. Breathe freely, keeping your chest open and your spine lengthened.

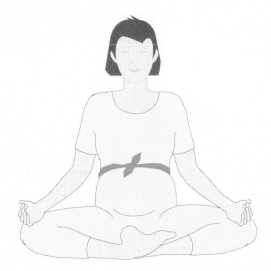

## CROSS-LEGGED POSE

Once your back is strengthened, you may attempt to sit in the cross-legged pose, which helps to straighten your spine. It is one of the most comfortable postures for the back and is easily attainable by most people. The triangular base provides increased stability for the rod-like spine. Try to lift the entire back upwards without accentuating the mid-spine arch.

1 Sit on the floor, initially with your back against a wall, and cross your legs. Place your hands on your knees with your palms up or down. The palms-up position can help to lift a heavy mind, which prevents the back from sinking too heavily into the floor. The palms-down position will help to ground you if you feel light-headed or are drifting off.

2 Finish the session by lying in the Corpse pose (see opposite) for at least 10 minutes.

pregnancy

## SUPINE CHAIR

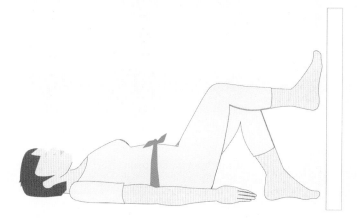

1 Lie down on your back, facing a wall, with your arms by your sides and your neck straight. Bend your knees, keeping your feet on the floor. Breathe in, raise your right foot and press it against the wall. Hold for a count of 10. Breathe out and lower your foot on to the floor. Now swap legs. Repeat 5 times on each side. On finishing, stretch out both legs for 5–12 breaths. Bend your knees and lower your feet to the floor.

## CORPSE POSE

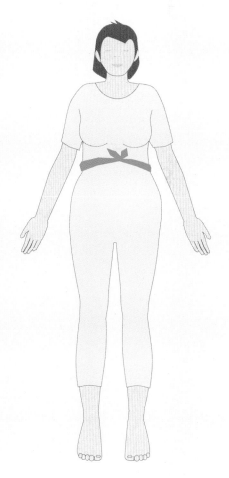

1 Lie on your back with feet apart and palms facing up. Breathe in and lower your chin. Breathe out slowly and allow your neck and shoulders to 'sink' towards the floor.

2 Take a deep breath in, lift your arms and stretch them out on the ground behind your head. Flex your toes to stretch the back of the legs. Breathe out slowly and relax. Go back to normal breathing. Lower your arms to your sides again.

3 Take a deep breath in and press your shoulders down away from your neck. Stretch your fingers out and point to your toes with your outstretched arms. Breathe out slowly and relax. Revert to observing normal breath.

4 Now breathe in and turn your head to the right so that your right ear is touching the floor. Keep your left shoulder pressed down to the floor. Maintain this stretch on breathing out. Go back to normal breathing. Relax the left side of your neck and shoulders, Stay in this position for 2–3 minutes. Repeat on the other side.

5 Now lie still. Keep your breathing below the ribcage. Relax your muscles completely. Lie like this for 20 minutes.

6 Slowly turn to the right with your right hand under your head. Relax, then roll over and repeat on the left.

## EMOTIONS

Here is an ancient saying:

*The baby eats what her mother eats, breathes what she does, thinks how she does, works when she does, rests when she does, emotes when she does, smiles when she does, cries when she does, hates when she does, loves when she does.*

Each of the emotions alters the state of the body and certainly affects the mind. The unborn baby cannot but react to its mother's state of mind. Stress, depression and anger all adversely affect your body, and learning to manage them will not only make your life easier now, it will help with bonding and bringing up your baby later.

■ As the Relaxation section of the Lifestyle Programme explains, relaxing is not simply doing nothing or sitting in front of the TV. Being able to consciously relax your muscles and switch off your mind will raise your threshold to stress. There will be times during pregnancy and the birth when you will feel worried or nervous, things may not go according to plan, you may feel out of control or that it is 'all too much'. Relaxation techniques are a tremendous help at these times.

■ You may find yourself more greatly affected by stressful situations or news than you would normally be; even events on the world stage or disaster movies can cause harmful agitation. Avoid them when you can.

■ Pregnancy yoga exercises will increase your mental as well as your physical stamina, and help your body react better to stress.

■ Exploring the spiritual side of life can expand the resources on which you can count. I personally feel that prayer can provide a lot of inner strength.

## HARMFUL SUBSTANCES

Smoking, alcohol and recreational drugs retard foetal growth. De-addict yourself before you get pregnant or do it as soon as you know about your pregnancy. Hypnosis, psychotherapy and acupuncture are very useful.

## SEX ADVICE

Although general advice is that you can continue to make love for as long as you are happy and comfortable doing so, I believe it is better to refrain from sex as far as possible. Sexual excitement brings turmoil to a woman's body when it should be in a state of calm. Where there has been a history of miscarriage the spasms of orgasm can cause damage, especially in the early and late stages of pregnancy, and so sex is best avoided during the first and third trimesters.

This is a time, however, to show a lot of mutual affection and love. Massage, sweet words, touches and embraces, gentle kisses and stroking are enjoyed best by women during pregnancy. And there are various ways a man can reach satisfaction without penetration. Talking through with your partner how you feel at different stages of your pregnancy is vital, so that there is no loss of mutual understanding and co-operation.

## UNNECESSARY STRAIN

This applies to both your muscles and your internal systems.

*Avoid:*

◆ sitting with your legs crossed. Sit with your feet firmly planted and your knees slightly apart – a little inelegant but better for you – or with legs flat and apart when sitting on the ground.

◆ straining on the toilet. If constipated, take psyllium husks or senna to ease the bowels.

◆ overhot baths.

◆ overdoing domestic chores. Enlist your partner or the rest of the family to do more than usual. Work in small spells, allowing yourself time to rest in between. Avoid carrying heavy things.

## Checks and check-ups

Once your pregnancy has been confirmed, you can expect to be called for regular check-ups to ensure your blood pressure and weight are staying within normal bounds, and to check that your baby is developing at the right rate.

You should also keep a regular check on yourself. Many women try to lead their lives as closely as possible to their pre-pregnant state, only their size forcing them to slow down in the final months. Take stock periodically, and regularly ask yourself questions such as:

◆ Am I getting enough good-quality sleep or is insomnia a problem?

◆ Is it time to give up work, or to arrange easier hours?

◆ Do I have the energy to do all the things I feel I am committed to? Should I set new priorities?

◆ Am I finding life more of a strain? This often shows in short temper, snappishness, fatigue and lack of concentration (ask your family and friends for their honest opinions).

◆ Am I allowing myself time to think about the future, planning the birth and my impending motherhood? Becoming a mother involves a fundamental change to your life, so it helps to begin making mental adjustments during your pregnancy.

## AMNIOCENTESIS

Amniocentesis is a procedure used to screen for genetic disorders such as Down's syndrome, thalassaemia (a blood disorder), cystic fibrosis and sickle cell anaemia. Because pregnancy carries higher risks in later life, particularly after the age of 40, amniocentesis is considered routine for older mothers-to-be.

The technique requires carrying out analysis of the amniotic fluid that surrounds the foetus, cushioning it from external injury. The fluid is collected during a precise surgical procedure that requires great expertise in order to minimize risk to the foetus.

Pregnant women who might undergo amniocentesis are presented with a dilemma. If the results are positive for a disorder that will seriously curtail a child's quality of life, should they have an abortion? (1 in 200 abortions may follow after the procedure, either through the parents' choice or because the surgical procedure itself can cause abortion.) If the decision would be to continue with the pregnancy irrespective of the result, then is it better to know, and so be prepared? Or is it better not to have the test, which carries an element of risk in itself? These are not easy decisions, but need to be considered before agreeing to the test.

# Common complaints during pregnancy Completely trouble-free pregnancies are very rare, but there are simple ways to alleviate some of the problems.

## MORNING SICKNESS

About half of pregnant women suffer from morning sickness (which can occur at any time of day) and it is most usual in the first trimester, between the second and twelfth weeks. It is typically worse with multiple pregnancies. The nausea and vomiting can be precipitated by the sight and smell of food, and can be made worse by emotional problems or anxiety about being pregnant.

It is believed that hormones secreted by the placenta may be responsible for morning sickness, as may redistribution of blood. With the depot of blood shifted to the lower abdomen, women with an existing history of neck tension or previous traumas may feel aware of an acute shortage of blood circulation in the head.

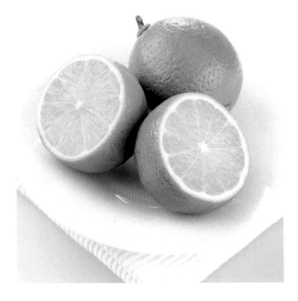

## What helps

With morning sickness, especially if it is severe, the last thing you will feel like doing is eating, but it is obviously important that you continue to get all the nourishment both you and your baby need, and at this time early in the pregnancy, the demand for food is high. The following should be helpful in overcoming the sense of nausea:

◆ a brief neck massage for 10 minutes or so first thing in the morning.
◆ putting a hot water bottle (wrapped in a towel) under your neck and lying on it for a while before getting up.
◆ gentle osteopathic manipulation once a week for the first few weeks of pregnancy.
◆ acupressure. On the inner surface of the arm, about three fingers above the wrist and in the middle, is an acupressure point called 'nei guan'. It is painful when pressed with the index finger or thumb of the opposite hand. Massaging and stimulating this point often helps to relieve nausea and sickness.
◆ the smell of fresh lime. Either use fresh lime or put a few drops of lime essential oil (lemon grass might work, too) on a tissue and sniff every few minutes.
◆ fresh air: open all windows to let in fresh air, and use an air purifier if you can.
◆ retention breathing (see page 74).

Although there are anti-nausea drugs available, these are usually only considered by doctors as a last resort. As Thalidomide tragically illustrated, drugs that are effective in what they are designed for can sometimes have terrible side-effects on a foetus.

## BACKACHE

Tension in the neck and tingling in the fingers in the early stage of pregnancy are mainly due to the dropping of the shoulders. In the later stages, as the abdomen bulges, low backache becomes a problem as the spine realigns itself to counteract the extra weight in front. The lower back (lumbar) muscles and buttocks come under great strain.

### What helps

*Yoga exercises*

Lie on your back. Bend your knees, keeping heels hip-distance apart. Lift your pelvis 15cm or so above the ground and hold for 5 seconds before lowering to the floor. Repeat 5–10 times.

Stand with your feet together. Tighten your buttocks. Place both hands on your buttocks, take a deep breath in and push your buttocks forwards. (Tightening your buttocks will prevent you from pushing your hips too far forward.) Don't bend your knees. Hold this position for 5 seconds. Breathe out as you return to the original position. Repeat 5 times.

*The groin factor*

I have been treating backache for over 20 years and have observed that the majority of lower backache stems from tenderness of the groin area, usually resulting from an injury (which can be caused by certain sorts of exercising, such as weights, tennis and squash, or kickboxing). The pain in the groin area makes the hips twist laterally or tilt forward, causing strain to the muscles in the lumbar region. Pregnancy creates this same sort of strain in the lower abdominal muscles, and the tendons above the pubic bone become sore on one side.

Locate this tender spot, on the right or left just above the pubic bone, and massage gently. Do not press hard or too deeply, as it is a very sore area. Massage the buttock on the same side.

*Massage*

Lie on your side with a pillow under your neck to support your head. Ask your partner to massage your neck and right down your spine, massaging just to either side of the centre of the spine.

## HIGH BLOOD PRESSURE

Your blood pressure will always be checked at routine prenatal check-ups, because high blood pressure could indicate a kidney problem or pre-eclampsia, a potentially dangerous condition (see page 169). If your blood pressure raises concern you may be told to rest completely or even be admitted to hospital. Since stress and diet contribute to high blood pressure, it is wise to take precautions to avoid reaching this stage.

### What helps

◆ eat less salt
◆ eat plenty of green vegetables, fruits and simple proteins such as chicken or fish, rather than red meat
◆ walk daily in a park or the countryside, breathing gently and slowly
◆ practise relaxation techniques
◆ stop working occasionally, to relax for a few minutes
◆ avoid over-thrilling or violent films
◆ refrain from too-frequent intercourse (perhaps once every 10 days). Excitement, especially unfulfilled, may cause a lot of tension. Gentle embracing, kissing and sensual massage, however, are beneficial
◆ aromatherapy and massage of your shoulders and neck (your partner may be able to do this for you).

Try using the above techniques first. A further step is homeopathy or herbal tinctures. Valerian drops on the tongue twice daily is helpful, but always consult a qualified integrated medical physician or homeopath first.

## VARICOSE VEINS AND HAEMORRHOIDS

The growing weight of the baby puts tremendous pressure on the veins in the lower part of the body. This is worse if the baby is large. The pressure causes congestion in the circulatory system, and the valves that control blood flow become non-functional. The result is varicose veins. Straining due to constipation and the downward pressure during labour similarly dilate the veins, leading to haemorrhoids (piles) or worsening varicose veins.

Tightness and cramping in the calves restricts the blood circulation through deeper veins and forces it through superficial veins, making them swell. This increases the risk of varicose veins.

### What helps
◆ Get your partner to massage your calves at bedtime with a massage oil – massage gently upwards from the ankle. If you do this from the beginning of your pregnancy, the channels of veins can be reduced.
◆ Keep your feet raised with a single pillow at night.
◆ Lie or sit in bed with your legs stretched out. Draw your ankles towards your body and hold them in this position for 5 counts. Then extend them as far as possible and hold in that position for 5 counts. This will stretch the muscles and skin of the legs. Do this 3–4 times a day.

Cramp or tightness in the calves can also be a sign of drinking too little water (or losing too much fluid through sweating), or a lack of minerals, particularly calcium. Constipation often leads to poor calcium absorption. Make sure you are not constipated:

◆ drink plenty of water (1½ to 2 litres per day)
◆ eat prunes, figs, spinach, beetroot, yoghurt, squash, okra
◆ if need be, use a gentle laxative such as syrup of figs or psyllium husks.

Haemorrhoids are much itchier or more painful when they protrude outside the rectum and become dry. Use a wet tissue to push them gently back into the rectum.

Lymphatic drainage massage (by a professional) is very beneficial in improving circulation in the lower limbs.

## INCONTINENCE OR TROUBLE URINATING

As the baby grows, the enlarging uterus presses on the bladder, reducing its capacity. In addition, the ligaments of the abdominal muscles get stretched and sore in the area where they are attached to the pubic bone. This may give the false sensation of an irritable bladder (rather like a urinary tract infection or cystitis), giving the urge to urinate frequently, even though the bladder is not full.

### What helps
◆ Massage the area above the pubic bone.
◆ Practise pelvic floor exercises (see page 211).

## BREAST TENDERNESS

At around six to eight weeks into the pregnancy, your breast are likely to become extremely tender, with sensations that can range from slight tingling to severe pain. This is primarily due to enlargement of the breast tissue in preparation for breastfeeding. Some secretions may take place through the nipples after 16 weeks.

### What helps
Massaging your breasts in the first few weeks of pregnancy will reduce pain later. Use cocoa butter, and massage from the outside towards the nipples. You may feel hard lumps – focus on these. Squeeze them gently between your thumb and fingers, as if kneading. Once they become slightly softer, they are less likely to hurt later.

When the actual tenderness and swelling starts, hot poultices might help. Heat together a cup of salt and 1 teaspoon of mustard seeds in a pan, then pour the salt in the centre of a handkerchief and tie up into a poultice. Wrap in another layer of hand towel or kitchen roll as it may be too hot. Apply this on the sore area. Do this in the morning and evening for five months or to relieve the congestion and pain.

## BREATHLESSNESS

In the later stages of pregnancy, the swelling abdomen cannot participate in breathing and the diaphragm cannot move very easily, so breathing becomes shallower, with the neck muscles helping pull the chest upwards. This leads to a certain amount of hyperventilation. A propensity to abdominal gas makes it even more difficult to breathe easily.

### What helps
Abdominal gas is caused by yeast overgrowth, fizzy water, constipation and high stomach acid. Keep to the dietary guidelines in the Lifestyle Programme to reduce this problem, allowing the diaphragm freer movement; this will make your breathing easier and more efficient.

Also practise controlled breathing: inhaling for 3 seconds, holding your breath for 3 seconds, breathing out slowly over 6 seconds.

## INDIGESTION AND HEARTBURN

The heartburn and reflux of stomach acid that are common complaints during pregnancy are generally due to excess stomach acid secretion. When the acidity level in the stomach is high, the stomach cannot empty its contents into the duodenum so quickly because it needs to wait for sufficient neutralizing bile to be produced.

The result is indigestion, gas, pain or discomfort. As the uterus grows in size, the stomach is somewhat squashed, which exacerbates matters.

### What helps
Avoid acid or sour foods, especially if you have a history of stomach ulcers, gastritis and heartburn.

## GALLSTONES

Bile can become thick and stagnant due to the pressure from the lower abdomen, and this can lead to the formation of gallstones.

### What helps
Regular exercise; control of abdominal gas with diet, by avoiding yeast, fizzy drinks and acidic food.

## UNUSUAL CRAVINGS

Your saliva reflects differing hormone levels in your blood and this can affect your sense of taste – many women find they have a distinct metallic taste in their mouth, which affects the flavour of food. In India, a woman eating pickles (particularly sour mango and lime pickles) is often a first outward sign of pregnancy in a culture discreet about mentioning such a condition. Pica, or the craving for odd things (coal, chalk, laundry starch or earthen pots are quite often reported), is sometimes believed to indicate an unconscious attempt to make up for a nutritional deficiency, such as calcium.

### What helps
Ensure you are getting all the nutrients you need (bearing in mind, for instance, that constipation can inhibit your absorption of calcium) and try to curb cravings for sweet foods or inedible substances.

## STRETCH MARKS

Stretch marks over the breasts and abdomen (you may also see them on your hips and upper arms) are mostly noticed after the birth, but reducing the effect should begin much earlier. These marks show red at first and then fade to look like faint irregular scars. They are not directly due to stretching but to the collagen in the skin being affected, reducing elasticity.

### What helps

Keep your skin well lubricated by massaging these areas with almond oil. If you are prone to them, stretch marks won't go away completely but the massage will help. Continue to massage after the baby is born, using ghee, almond oil or mustard oil to nourish the skin and restore its lost elasticity.

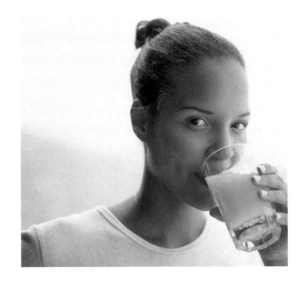

## CHLOASMA

Some women are alarmed to find chloasma, or 'the mask of pregnancy', is darkening the skin over their forehead and across their nose and cheekbones. It happens more often in women with darker skin, and is the result of increased melanin production – the same mechanism that causes your skin to tan in the sun and, in pregnancy, darkens the nipples and makes visible the linea nigra down your abdomen. It fades after the birth.

### What helps

Exposure to the sun increases melanin production, so avoid too much sunbathing and use a high-factor sun cream on your face.

As chloasma is an indication that the adrenal glands are overactive, exercise and stress management can help restore the balance, as can neck massage.

## GUM PROBLEMS

A softening and slight sponginess of the gums is quite usual in pregnancy, and not an indication of tooth decay. (But do continue to visit your dentist for regular check-ups.)

### What helps

Lack of vitamin C or calcium may cause some swelling in the gums and bleeding, so ensure you are getting sufficient of these nutrients.

## EXCESSIVE SALIVATION

Excessive salivation is not so common, but is a troublesome complaint. It may be associated with morning sickness or, later, be linked with increased appetite.

### What helps

Homoeopathic remedies are good: try belladonna 30 tablets, 3 times a day.

# Exercises to improve circulation in the legs

Sit with your legs stretched out in front of you. Keeping your knees straight, flex your feet forwards and then upwards, stretching your toes back towards you as far as possible. Hold for 5 seconds. Repeat 20 times, twice a day.

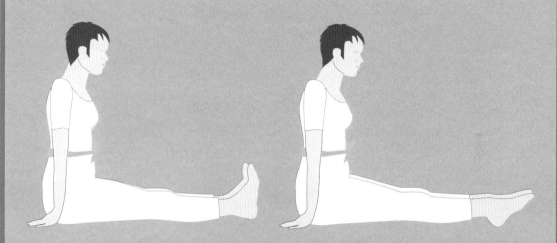

Lie on your back. Lift one leg and bend the foot at the ankle 5–10 times as above. Repeat with the other leg.

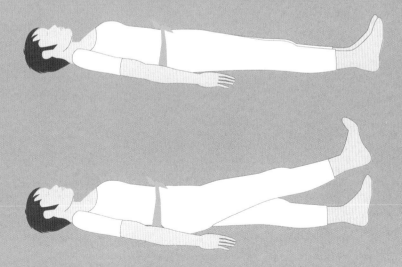

# Problems that can arise Some of the following are common and only problematic if left unchecked; others are potentially serious (but usually rare).

## BLOOD CLOTS

Haemorrhaging is a serious threat to pregnancy and so, as a safeguard, the blood increases its clotting power. But a greater tendency to clot brings its own problems, in the form of possible thrombosis.

### What helps
The liver is responsible for regulating various clotting factors, but when oestrogen levels rise during pregnancy, this puts pressure on the functions of the liver (which also metabolizes oestrogen). Avoid anything that puts further strain on the liver: alcohol, fried food, cheese, excess butter and yeast products (yeast causes gut fermentation, producing alcohols that affect the liver).

## ANAEMIA

Many women are very slightly anaemic, and being pregnant increases the demand for iron. Iron, along with protein, folic acid and trace elements such as cobalt, is vital to the synthesis of haemoglobin.

### What helps
Although your body adjusts by absorbing nutrients more efficiently in pregnancy, you may be getting too little iron in your diet. Red meat, eggs, spinach, seeds and liver (but see box) are all good sources. But eating plenty of iron is not enough if your stomach lining cannot do its job efficiently. Avoid acidic foods that can irritate your stomach and cause digestive problems. Supplementation may be necessary if the dietary sources are not enough.

## THE LIVER CONTROVERSY

In general, foods that help blood synthesis (protein, iron, folic acid) are also recommended for infertility and pregnancy. The controversy arises with liver. Since liver stores vitamin A, which in experimental mice causes abortion, it is banned for pregnant women. In a newspaper column, I once recommended liver for anaemic pregnant women and scores of emails from doctors and practitioners bombarded my office.

I only spoke of what was traditionally recommended, and believe the confusion lies in the difference between vitamin A from natural dietary sources and vitamin A in supplementary form, as a tablet or capsule.

If you eat a lot of liver, it will go through your digestive system and any vitamin A excess to your body's requirements will be stored in your own liver. Concentrated vitamin A in medicinal form, however, is designed to be absorbed straight away and forcefully enter the bloodstream, and therein lies the danger.

You should therefore not take vitamin A supplements, but I do recommend liver once a week to pregnant women, especially if there is a tendency to anaemia. However, do bear in mind that this is just an option. You can take iron, protein, $B_{12}$ and pomegranate (for cobalt) if you don't like liver.

## THAI BASIL

Thai basil helps circulation and promotes relaxation. It is available in oriental or Thai grocery shops, and some supermarkets. Add basil leaves to soup and sauces. Make a basil leaf tea by infusing a few leaves in hot water for about 5 minutes and then straining. Add a little honey.

- soft-boiled eggs
- porridge
- home-made chicken soup
- puréed or soft-cooked vegetables
- pomegranates, bananas
- 'soft' meals such as shepherd's pie or pasta with a minced meat sauce
- boil prawns in their shells for 1 hour – use the stock and prawns to make a soothing soup.

### BLEEDING

About 20 per cent of women experience some bleeding in the first trimester. This is usually without cramping. The exact cause of this bleeding is not known but it is attributed to the implantation of the embryo or the formation of the placenta irritating the lining of the uterus.

#### What helps

For bleeding in early pregnancy and small bleeding in advanced pregnancy, seek help immediately. Strict bed rest is absolutely necessary. Use a low pillow and lie mostly on your back. Get up only to go to the toilet, not even for a bath – for two or three days limit yourself to a bed bath with a sponge – until the bleeding shows no sign of restarting. Enhance your ability to relax by:

- listening to pleasant music and relaxation tapes
- staying calm (even discourage energetic friends from calling, to avoid over-excitement). When your heart rate is lower this aids clotting, so the bleeding stops
- neck massage (while still on your back)
- reflexology
- sniffing rose or lavender oil.

Adjust your diet to help your recovery and avoid recurrent bleeding. Eat easily digestible foods:

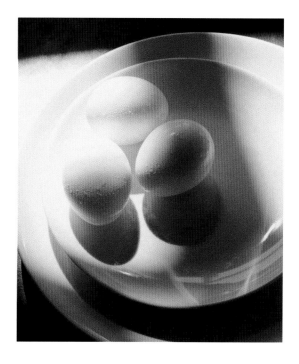

*Drink:*
- fresh fruit juices
- herbal teas (peppermint, chamomile, green tea).

*Avoid altogether:*
- alcohol
- coffee
- salty foods
- fizzy water.

## POOR GROWTH OF THE FOETUS

There are various reasons why a foetus does not grow according to expectations, especially in the first trimester. Keeping yourself healthy should prevent any worries, but bad morning sickness, loss of appetite, not resting enough and excessive physical activity are some of the commonest causes for anxiety about the growth of a baby. You will be checked to see that you are not suffering from a digestive disorder such as ulcerative colitis, Crohn's disease or chronic diarrhoea, which will cause malabsorption, interrupting foetal growth.

### What helps
Change your lifestyle straight away, to ensure that everything goes right from now on for you and your baby.

*Rest:*
Conserve your energy. You may need to stop work for at least three or four months to give your baby a chance to develop better. Take gentle walks, enjoy the garden or the park, but avoid strenuous exercise.

*Diet:*
- Eat plenty, concentrating on high-protein foods, sustaining carbohydrates (don't resort to creamy cakes and fried foods to put on weight) and vitamin- and mineral-packed food.
- Make chicken soup (see page 65) with cooked lentils. Drink this about 1½ hours before a main meal so that your appetite has returned by meal time – the soup is additional to your usual meals, not instead of them, so don't fill your stomach with soup and say you are full.
- Help your digestion by cooking fish, meat and vegetables with garlic, onions, and spices or herbs such as ginger, black pepper, thyme, rosemary, sage, dill.

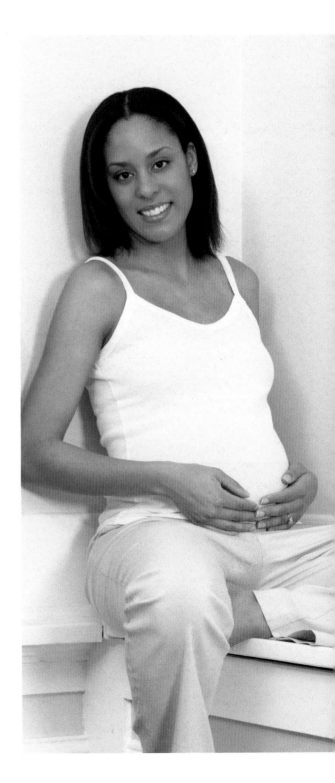

◆ Mince meat and purée vegetables to make them more easily digested.

◆ Add butter or ghee to lentils or rice.

◆ Avocado is nutritious and is a good source of non-dairy, non-saturated fats for strict vegetarians.

◆ Juice carrots and apples for a nutrient-filled drink.

◆ Pasta, rice, potatoes and soda bread are all sustaining carbohydrates.

◆ Snack on cottage cheese mixed with a teaspoonful of honey, almonds (soaked for 24 hours) or walnuts.

◆ If you are a strict vegetarian, talk to a qualified nutritionist about how best to improve your protein and vitamin/mineral intake.

*Supplements:*

◆ Take multivitamins with minerals; in particular you may need iron and folic acid.

◆ If you are vegetarian you will probably need to supplement your diet with protein powders or drinks recommended for pregnant women.

## PRE-ECLAMPSIA AND ECLAMPSIA

Eclampsia is a serious complication of pregnancy, fortunately occurring only in 0.5 per cent of all births. The exact cause is not known. The signs, usually in the final days of pregnancy, are very high blood pressure, seizures or fits, protein in the urine, abdominal pain, swelling of hands, feet and face, headaches, nausea, blurred vision and then lack of consciousness. Immediate hospitalization and delivery is required for this life-threatening condition.

Full-blown eclampsia is so rare because doctors are well aware of the warning signs and can take preventive action. Pre-eclampsia is signalled by high blood pressure accompanied by swelling of the extremities and protein in the urine. It is more frequent in women with a previous history of kidney problems.

**What helps**

If the blood pressure is not too high and the swelling not intense, then the following regime may be useful and hospitalization avoided.

The swelling (and also any protein in your urine) is related to your kidneys not functioning as well as they should. Be kind to them by:

◆ keeping your salt intake low

◆ drinking plenty of water

◆ drinking no coffee or alcohol

◆ drinking nettle and gokhru teas to help alleviate fluid retention.

Protein intake should be high (though check with your doctor first), and eat plenty of foods that are filling but not fattening, such as:

◆ vegetable soup made with chicken stock, with added lentils or rice

◆ beansprouts with grated ginger, spring onions and a few drops of lemon

◆ grilled vegetables.

Reduce tension and stress, and so help your blood pressure by:

◆ massaging neck and shoulder while lying on your side

◆ breathing exercises and relaxation techniques

◆ drink peppermint or chamomile tea

◆ mix 10–15 Valerian drops in half a cup of water, and drink twice daily.

Your doctor or health visitor will need to monitor your progress carefully and frequently, so that if the symptoms get worse they can act quickly.

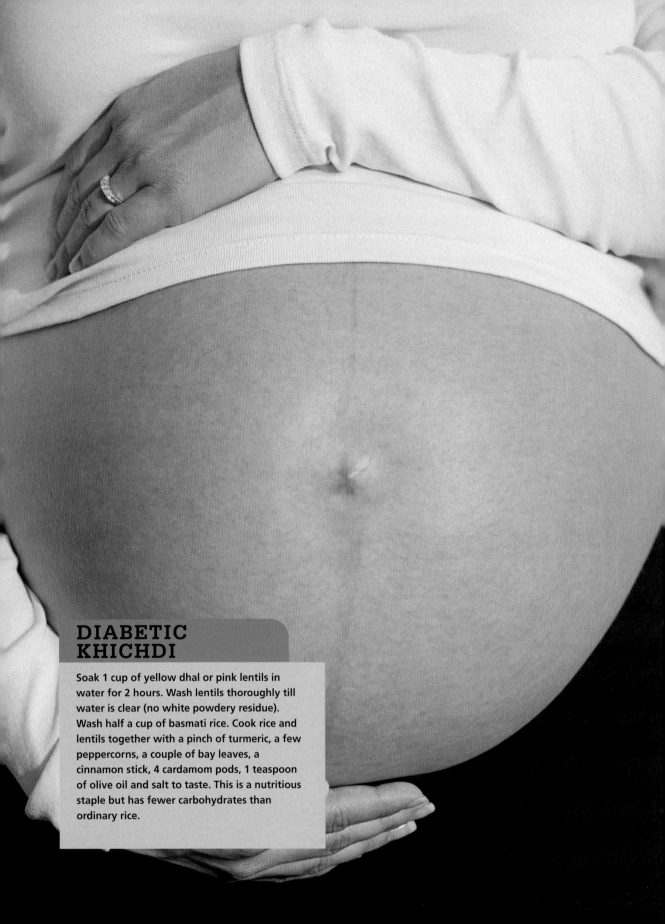

## DIABETIC KHICHDI

Soak 1 cup of yellow dhal or pink lentils in water for 2 hours. Wash lentils thoroughly till water is clear (no white powdery residue). Wash half a cup of basmati rice. Cook rice and lentils together with a pinch of turmeric, a few peppercorns, a couple of bay leaves, a cinnamon stick, 4 cardamom pods, 1 teaspoon of olive oil and salt to taste. This is a nutritious staple but has fewer carbohydrates than ordinary rice.

## GESTATIONAL DIABETES

Diabetes can occur during pregnancy and may or may not spontaneously disappear after the baby is born. The first signs are excessive thirst and frequent urination. This is one of the possible problems that are looked for in regular antenatal check-ups.

### What helps

Try first to treat gestational diabetes by diet and some exercises.

*Diet:*

You will need to balance your diet carefully to control your blood sugar levels. Your physician or health visitor will advise you on how to do this, but below is an example.

**Breakfast:** Poached or boiled eggs or cottage cheese, 10 almonds (soaked for 24 hours and then peeled), milk tea (i.e. made with all milk not water) or dandelion coffee added to hot milk.

**Lunch or dinner:** Green salad, vegetables (no potatoes or high-sugar, high-starch vegetables such as sweet potato or parsnips), chicken, turkey or fish with a small portion of plain pasta, bowl of low-starch rice or diabetic khichdi (see box opposite).

**Drink:** Herbal teas without added sugar. (Fruit teas have natural fructose.)

*Exercise:*

◆ Go for walks and practise the pregnancy yoga regime.
◆ Your physician or health visitor will continue to check your blood sugar levels regularly and if necessary give insulin injections.

## MISCARRIAGE

Miscarriage with a first pregnancy is a surprisingly common occurrence. The majority of miscarriages happen in the first trimester, and often very early on, and many women are not even aware they have miscarried.

Although most women go on to have successive safe and healthy pregnancies, repeated miscarriages do happen. Reasons for this include infection, a hormonal, immunological or genetic problem, malnutrition or a physical problem with the uterus or cervix. (You may hear the expression 'incompetent cervix': this means that the cervix cannot retain the foetus in place and it slips down into the vagina; the solution is to use stitches to hold the cervix closed until shortly before birth.)

The most usual sign of miscarriage, or threatened miscarriage, is bleeding, so any bleeding in pregnancy must be checked out straight away. If the bleeding is accompanied by lower backache and cramps, and the cervix has opened, then miscarriage is usually inevitable.

A later miscarriage, after the first trimester, can be more complicated. Sometimes the foetus dies but remains in the uterus. Women often sense it: their pulse is no longer fast, any food cravings disappear and their skin changes; they just don't 'feel pregnant' any longer. If you have any sense of this, don't wait for your next appointment, but go to see your doctor, who will check for a foetal heartbeat and possibly do an ultrasound scan.

Miscarrying, especially if you have had time to adjust to the idea of being pregnant and have begun to look forward to having a baby, is going to be traumatic. It is always good to spend a little time on your own initially, as comforting words from others, however well meant, might make matters worse. You may then seek the moral and emotional support of those close to you.

Give yourself time to recover, both physically and mentally. Take time off; take a relaxing holiday. Walking, yoga, meditation and relaxation techniques will all help ease your recovery time.

# Preparing for the birth Remember that not every woman experiences childbirth in the same way, and your experience will be personal to you.

## HOW THE BABY MOVES

In the late stages of pregnancy, hormones produce another remarkable change. The parathyroid glands secrete calcitonin, which increases the secretion of calcium. Areas like the pubic joints and the sacro-iliac joints in the lower back area become starved of calcium. This natural osteoporosis enables the entire pelvic girdle to unlock and increase in diameter, allowing the baby's head to descend into the pelvic region.

As the time for birth approaches, the baby shifts position. It tilts down head first and the head 'engages' in the pelvic girdle. Sometimes the baby fails to turn automatically, or half-turns, into what is called a breech position. An experienced midwife can often gently manipulate and turn the baby. Alternatively, acupuncture or moxibustion (using heat on acupuncture points) can prove beneficial, encouraging the uterine muscles to relax and allow gravity to do its job. Resting and relaxing helps the process; the more anxious you are, the more tense the uterine muscles will be, immobilizing the unborn baby.

## PLANNING THE BIRTH

Visit the maternity ward of your hospital, so that it is familiar to you, and ask about what facilities are available – it is no good setting your heart on a water birth and only discovering as you go into labour that there is no suitable pool or bath or no one experienced to assist you.

It is never possible to foresee exactly how a birth will proceed – it may take much longer than you imagine or

you may find your intention to use only natural pain relief goes out the window when the contractions are in full force. Talk to your gynaecologist or midwife about your options and the pros and cons of different types of birth, about delivery positions, about pain control, about the use of forceps and other aids. Raise any concerns you have as early as possible so that when labour begins everyone knows your preferences and you can feel as relaxed as possible about the process. You might like to write these down, so that everyone is clear about your wishes.

Having familiar faces with you through the birth is comforting and reassuring. There are differing views on whether this should include your partner. The current trend is for the father to be at the birth, but neither he nor you should feel pressurized into conforming to this fashion. If he has been accompanying you to antenatal classes, has been actively involved and well prepared in what to expect, then being present at the birth itself can be highly beneficial emotionally and good for bonding. But even then many men feel overwhelmed, helpless at being unable to assist and not the towering support either of you had envisaged. Many women find an experienced sister or close friend of greater practical support and this would be my own recommendation.

Discuss this with your partner beforehand, as it is important that he doesn't feel sidelined or excluded. His support is vital even if it doesn't include holding your hand through the birth itself.

Books can only prepare you to a certain extent and are no substitute for the actual experience of midwives and women who have been through it themselves. Take advantage of the wealth of experience at antenatal classes.

## THE INDIAN DAIS

There used to be a school in the ancient city of Varanasi, on the banks of the Ganges, where dais or midwives received practical training in the art of delivering babies and perinatal care of mother and child. They would arrive at a woman's home shortly before the delivery time and spend 40 days there after delivery, massaging, bathing, feeding, dressing, early-morning exposure to sunlight and cleaning the newborn, and massaging and advising the mother. The mother's primary role was to rest and breastfeed. If she was a first-time mother, she learnt how to take care of her baby and treat it for minor ailments. A few such dais still exist, employed by wealthy traditional families, but it is an art being lost, which is a pity. Hospital birth is common and such old-fashioned methods have been discarded in favour of the pediatrician or nurses.

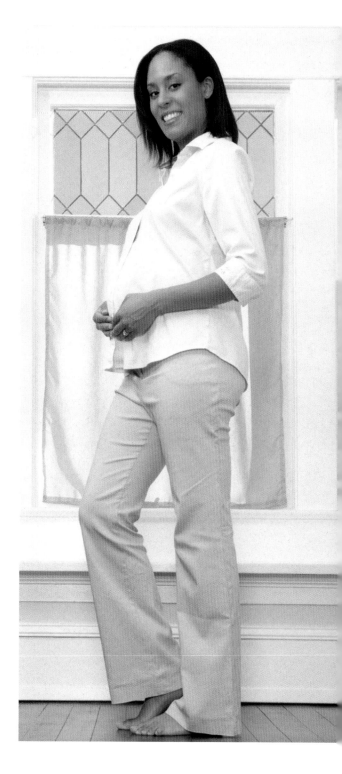

## THE LAST WEEK

For the last week before the baby is expected, get plenty of rest, and have your neck and shoulders massaged regularly to reduce stress and improve pituitary function.

*Include the following in your diet:*

◆ soft, easily digested food, such as mushy rice, porridge, soft-boiled eggs, minced meat/fish, soft-cooked vegetables
◆ carrots + apple + celery juice
◆ vegetable juice flavoured with saffron and honey
◆ pomegranates, pears, water chestnuts, yams and avocados
◆ small amounts of butter or ghee in lentil soup or steamed rice
◆ plenty of water.

## LABOUR

Early signs of labour include pain in the thighs, an urge to urinate and defecate (but with little result), restlessness, increased heart rate, and maybe sweating may increase. As the oestrogen level from the placenta rises, the uterine muscles become more susceptible to contraction. Another hormone, oxytocin, increases the contractions to a point of no return. (Obstetricians often use a synthetic form of this hormone to stimulate labour when contractions are weak or when labour has gone on too long.)

Minor pains towards the end of gestation do not necessarily indicate the onset of labour. With the uterine walls so stretched they may contract spontaneously, and many women have rushed to hospital only to find it was a false alarm.

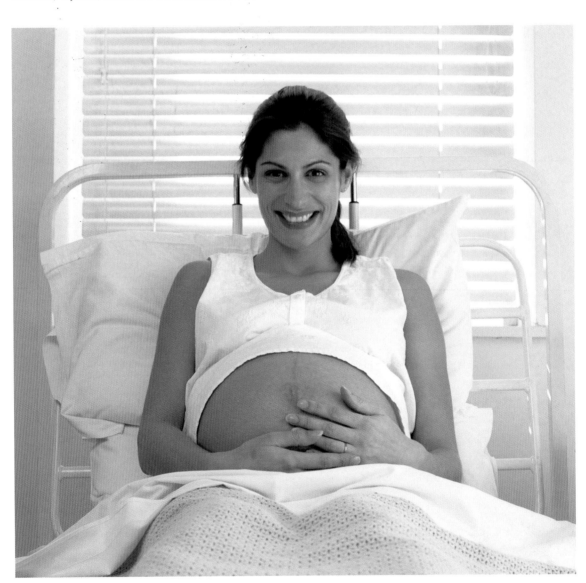

### Stages of labour

During labour the contractions begin at the top of the uterus and sweep down, like waves. These contractions occur at regular intervals and as birth progresses, they become stronger and more prolonged as the baby is pushed down. There are three stages of labour:

◆ dilation stage. The cervix (neck of the uterus) dilates completely and the baby moves into the cervical canal. The contractions occur at 10–30-minute intervals and last for 30 seconds or so. This stage can last eight hours, and is usually shorter with second and subsequent births. At the end of this stage the waters break (which means that the amniotic sac breaks, rather like a balloon bursting, and the fluid gushes out).

◆ expulsion stage. As the baby emerges, the head can be seen at the vaginal opening. Contractions occur every 2–3 minutes. This stage may be very short or last up to about 1½ hours. (If it goes on much longer than this, there may be a need to help the baby emerge, perhaps with forceps or ventouse.) The end of this stage is the birth itself.

◆ placental stage. The contractions continue until the placenta is expelled from the uterus, which happens within an hour of delivery. (The ½ litre of blood loss at this stage may seem alarming, but is quite usual, and the extra blood that you have had in your system during pregnancy means that you can easily sustain this loss.)

In theory, muscular spasm can cut off the blood supply to the endometrium. (When the contraction occurs, the small blood vessels that run through the myometrium to the endometrium are constricted, depriving the placenta of an adequate blood supply.) Because of this (the result of intense and frequent contractions during labour) the heart rate of the foetus increases, as its blood supply through the placenta is reduced.

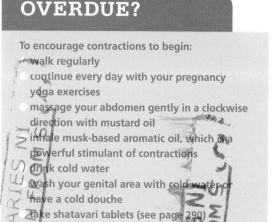

## OVERDUE?

To encourage contractions to begin:
- walk regularly
- continue every day with your pregnancy yoga exercises
- massage your abdomen gently in a clockwise direction with mustard oil
- inhale musk-based aromatic oil, which is a powerful stimulant of contractions
- drink cold water
- wash your genital area with cold water or have a cold douche
- take shatavari tablets (see page 290)

Useful aids are also to be found in acupuncture and homeopathy.

### Conserving your strength during labour

Rest is very important. Women who are more rested and relaxed find the contractions and birth easier to bear; labour is more difficult for tired and anxious mothers.

In the early stages of labour, when contractions are less frequent, head and neck massage by a supportive relative or partner, reflexology on your feet and similar relaxants are very beneficial. If you manage to sleep for an hour or so, you will wake up with greater energy and your muscles will contract better.

Food and drink during labour should be restricted to fluids, soups or fruit juice (such as apple, pomegranate, grape), but if the labour is long, some easily digestible food will give you renewed energy. Be prepared with something like soft-boiled eggs, fishcakes, oat biscuits, or a mushy dish such as mashed potato, dhal or porridge.

## ROMAN LAW

Contrary to popular belief, the term Caesarean has nothing to do with the birth of Julius Caesar. It is derived from lex Caesarea, the Roman law which decreed that before the burial of a woman who died in the late stages of pregnancy, the child must be removed with a cut to open her belly (caesum). Galen, the great Greek surgeon-physician to three consecutive Caesars, was the first to have performed this surgery to deliver babies in emergencies.

### Caesarean or C section

Delivering a baby by surgical incision into the uterus rather than following through a vaginal delivery can be a life-saving procedure in an emergency. However, it is estimated that some 15–20 per cent of deliveries are now Caesarean, which is almost certainly much higher than necessary. Convenience and fashion play a part in these statistics which vary from hospital to hospital. Situations where a Caesarean may be necessary include:

◆ placenta praevia, when the placenta is lying between the baby and the cervix and there is a threat of massive haemorrhage because the placenta will be delivered first, severing the baby's blood supply.
◆ foetal distress, perhaps from a very prolonged labour or a technicality such as the placenta separating from the wall of the uterus or the umbilical cord threatening to strangle the baby.
◆ the baby in a breech position that cannot be turned.
◆ multiple births (although a Caesarean is not always necessary with twins).
◆ an abnormally narrow pelvis or extra-large head (less usual than you might think).
◆ eclampsia (see page 169).
◆ uncontrollable phobia or fear in the mother.

Some mothers-to-be believe that a Caesarean will be less painful, less traumatic and avoid a stretched vagina or an episiotomy (cutting the skin around the vagina), but it is a mistake to think that a Caesarean is an easy option. Recovery from a Caesarean is slower and more painful, there is a greater risk of infection or postnatal complications and some mothers have found it more difficult to form a close bond with their new baby, especially if the operation was done under general anaesthetic. It has also been noticed that an unstressful vaginal birth is beneficial to the baby as well, somehow acting as a stimulant to facing life. The baby's immune system is usually better (fewer allergies, colds, etc.), he or she will suffer fewer headaches and be less prone to hyperactivity.

It is also a myth to think that if you have had one Caesarean delivery, all subsequent ones should be. Indeed, unless specifically indicated, it would be preferable to choose a vaginal birth after a Caesarean.

## Premature birth

In theory, a full-term baby is born at 38 weeks (40 weeks after your last period), but due dates are not always precise. A baby arriving a week or two early is not usually going to suffer any problems of prematurity.

Medical care for babies has developed to the stage where it is possible to save a baby born as early as 23 or 24 weeks, but such babies need an enormous amount of intensive care and do not always survive. Medical ability in this area is improving all the time, but the main difficulty remains, that a premature baby's lungs are insufficiently developed, and do not allow it to take in sufficient oxygen. However, these days the survival rate of premature babies treated in special care baby units is very good.

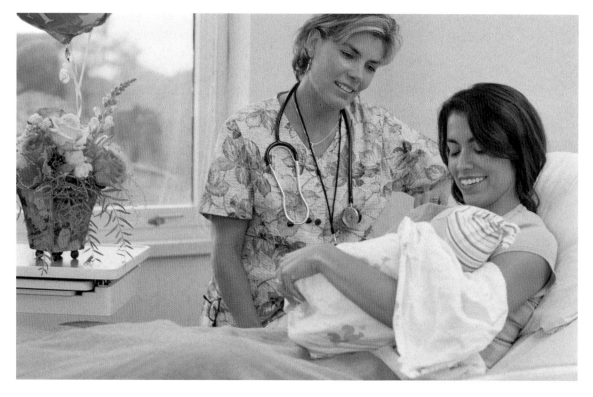

# After the birth

The joy of seeing and holding your new baby overrules everything, but labour is an exhausting business. You should be encouraged to sleep. Arrange to have the following ready, to help your rest and recuperation in the hours following the birth:

◆ grape or apple juice, freshly squeezed if possible. Other cold drinks are useful to help calm down a tired body

◆ drink a ginger and fennel infusion 3–4 times a day; boil 1 tsp of fennel seeds with 1 tsp grated ginger for 10 minutes, then leave to cool

◆ massage for the soles of the feet with a soothing cream or oil

◆ home-made chicken soup, for replenishing but easily digested sustenance (see page 65).

*Supplements:*

These will all help restore energy and give you a sense of well-being.

◆ shatavari

◆ kolonji or black cumin seed oil (Nigella sativa)

◆ multivitamins and minerals

◆ chawanprash and shilajit (ayurvedic supplements).

# A new mother

Pregnancy is not an end in itself, it is just the beginning. In the next chapter I look at important aspects of a new mother's health, coping with feeding a newborn baby, recovering from the strains of pregnancy and labour, and finding her feet in a changed life.

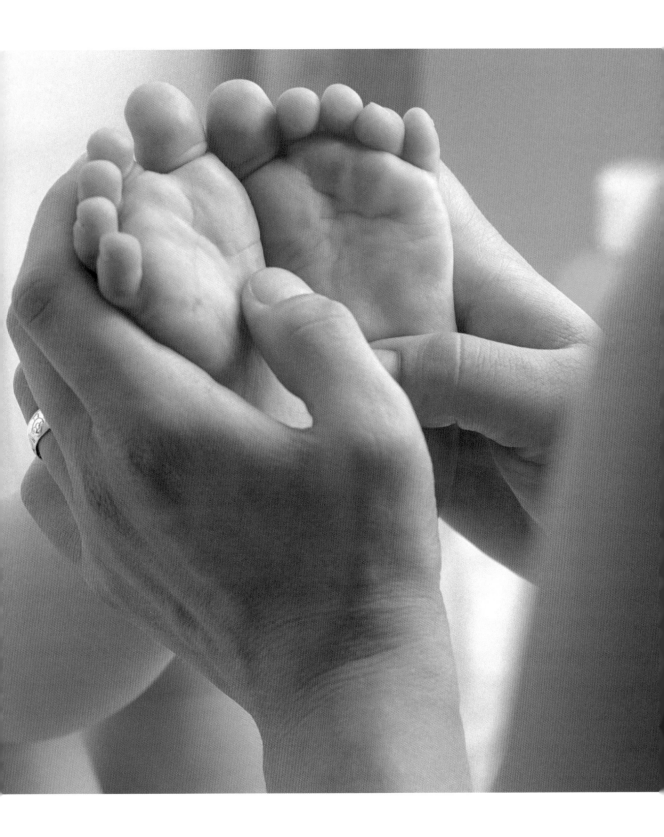

# chapter four

# a new mother

Caring for a newborn baby is a very demanding job. In a traditional extended family, a young mother would have helped care for younger relatives, and could rely on a host of experienced mothers to help and give her advice. The typical situation nowadays is very different and, however much you may have read about the theory of baby care, the reality can come as a shock. But this book is primarily about your health, as a new mother. After all, your own health and your baby's are inextricably linked, so your well-being in these early days is vital. The healthier you are, the better for your baby – if you are relaxed, your baby is more likely to be too. And the healthier and happier your baby, the less strain there is on you.

# The shock of the new

From the point of view of the baby, being born is quite a shocking experience: the pressure in the birth canal with the strong contractions squeezing body and head, the emergence from a world of darkness into the brightness of the labour room, the brief pause before that first gasp of air is taken in to fill the lungs for the first time. What a baby needs most now is enveloping warmth and reassurance.

In a home birth this is just what a new baby would be given – a wash and initial check-up, then wrapping warmly and being placed in the mother's arms – and most hospitals now follow this practice, rather than removing the baby to a nursery. The argument for separating mother and baby was to allow the mother to rest, and while it is true that you will probably be exhausted, it is not the baby who is going to tire you in the first days, but too many visitors and general over-excitement. Simply cuddling your baby quietly will work wonders for both of you.

# Forging bonds
Bonding starts while you are still pregnant, but it is not automatic. Don't feel discouraged or inadequate if your first feeling is not a huge rush of maternal affection.

At last you have your baby in your arms, the moment you have been waiting for for nine months. For many women there is an instant bond from the first second they hold their child. However, if you were ambivalent about being pregnant in the first place, or had a difficult labour, or if your new baby is not well and has to be kept in an incubator, or even if your nature is just to take things cautiously, you may find it takes more time and patience to build up a bond between you.

If this is your first child you may feel out of your depth. Everyone else will seem to be more confident and to know more (even if their advice is conflicting). Without meaning to, busy nursing staff, bossy mothers and even overbearing partners can make you feel the baby is less 'yours', and slow down that crucial feeling of bonding.

Like friendships, true bonds grow stronger as you get to know each other. Cuddle and touch your baby as often as possible. Skin-to-skin contact brings comfort on both sides, and stroking, hugging, kissing and breastfeeding are all important to building up a loving relationship. And the more you get to recognize little signs, different cries, the easier it will be for you to fulfil your baby's needs and the more contented your baby will be.

## Massage

All babies who are massaged regularly are healthier for it. Massaging is healing and improves circulation, which means better nourishment for your baby's body and brain. It is also a perfect way to make your child feel loved, pampered and cared for.

*Massage also has other advantages.*

◆ Babies who are massaged regularly develop well and the milestones that are usually used to measure this development (crawling, sitting, etc.) tend to appear slightly earlier than predicted in childcare books.
◆ Babies have fewer colds and coughs, as massaging stimulates their immune system.
◆ They also sleep much better during the day and certainly at night.

There is no special technique to massaging your baby, but here's how the dais, or midwives, would go about it in a traditional Indian home:

> They would begin to massage the baby once it was five days old. They would massage the neck, back, arms and legs with a little oil, toning up the muscles. In winter they would use a 'warming' mustard oil diluted with sesame, and during the summer a lighter coconut oil. After six months, they would gently include the head, ears and jaw. The baby would then be put in the sun for up to half an hour.

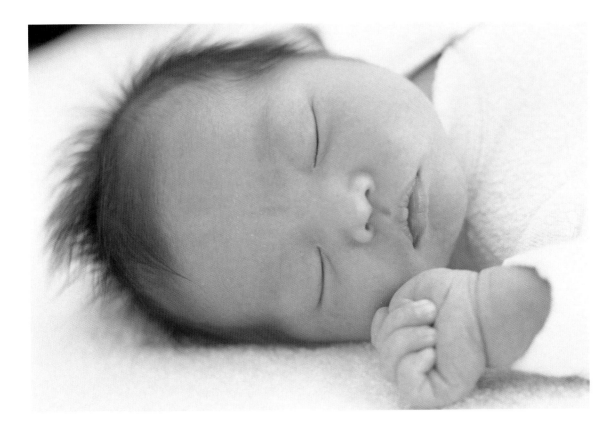

## CRANIAL OSTEOPATHY

This is a specialized form of osteopathy that has a particular application for young babies. Labour puts tremendous pressure on all parts of the body, especially when the labour is short (under 2 hours) or very long (over 20 hours). A newborn's face and skull can be quite distorted by the delivery, as the bones of the skull are not joined together, but these soon realign themselves before fusing. By making minute adjustments to these bones, cranial osteopaths aim to improve circulation of the cerebrospinal fluid that bathes the brain and nourishes it.

If you lubricate your hands with a light oil, such as baby oil, and just gently rub and knead your baby's body all over, it will prove a thoroughly enjoyable and beneficial experience for you both, and you will soon learn what gets a happy response. The exposure to the sun that the dais practised allowed the skin to synthesize vitamin D, which ensures better absorption of calcium. This is an essential mineral in a growing baby, particularly for bones and muscle movement, so you might like to follow this example.

About once a week dais would give a baby a short dunk in cold water to 'shock' the system, wrapping the baby up immediately afterwards. This is called 'tempering' and was used in Greek and Roman times as well. This makes the body tougher, to cope with sudden chills.

# Breastfeeding

Some women take very naturally to breastfeeding, their baby suckles easily, the milk supply is satisfying and they find the experience of nursing an enjoyable one that helps them bond with their new son or daughter.

For other women, things are not so easy. The milk doesn't always flow well to begin with; cracked and sore nipples or the heaviness of the breasts can be painful; there may be too little milk to satisfy a demanding infant. In addition, breastfeeding on demand, particularly at night, is extremely tiring, and moving to an alternative as soon as possible seems very tempting.

Lack of confidence, conflicting advice and painful or unsuccessful early attempts put a lot of women off breastfeeding, which leads to further anxiety as they feel they are 'failing', and persevering becomes an additional pressure among many others.

## Why is breastfeeding a good idea?

Breast milk is the ideal first food for a baby for several reasons.

◆ It is easy to digest and absorb.
◆ Antibodies in mother's milk help prevent infections before a baby's own immune system has developed fully – breastfed babies suffer less from common ailments such as coughs, colds, diarrhoea and tummy cramps (provided the mother eats well).
◆ Breast milk provides greater protection from allergies – fewer breastfed children are troubled by allergic reactions such as asthma.

◆ Breastfed babies are inclined to sleep better and be more content.
◆ It is more hygienic and convenient than mixing formula milk and sterilizing bottles.
◆ Once mastered, it is an enjoyable way of bonding for both mother and child.

In many parts of the world, breastfeeding continues for many months, even a year or so. Yet in the UK fewer than 50 per cent of mothers breastfeed for over six weeks. That average is the lowest in Europe. Typical reasons for not breastfeeding, or giving up early, include:

◆ not 'getting the hang of it'
◆ not producing sufficient milk to satisfy the baby
◆ milk supply drying up
◆ discomfort from neck ache or backache while feeding
◆ painful or cracked nipples
◆ painfully heavy, engorged or saggy breasts
◆ worry about losing figure.

All these except the last are valid complaints, but they are usually avoidable and comparatively few women cannot breastfeed successfully, and for at least six months. This is not something that necessarily comes naturally, and too often first-time mothers are given insufficient advice and come to the conclusion, wrongly, that they are not cut out for breastfeeding. The last reason is actually a misconception (see page 191).

# A happy experience

Understanding the mechanisms of milk production and flow is useful (see box), and the following practical tips should also prove helpful.

## ENCOURAGING A GOOD MILK SUPPLY

### Nursing positions

Enlist the help of your midwife or an experienced friend or family member to advise or demonstrate:

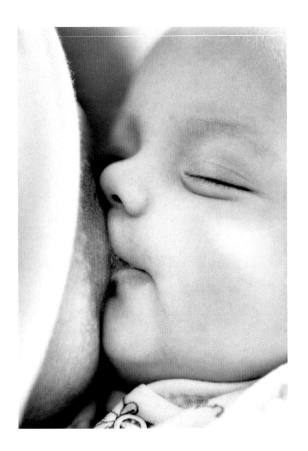

- ways to hold your baby while breastfeeding. If you are uncomfortable or are straining back or arm muscles, your baby will be ill at ease too. Try out different props with cushions and pillows. A pillow or two on your lap will raise your baby up and take some of the weight from your arms. Try out ideas before the birth, as for the first days afterwards you will be both busy and tired and less keen to learn and experiment.

## MILK FLOW

It is often assumed that a baby simply extracts the milk from the breasts by suction, but the reality is more subtle than that. As new mothers have found, simply hearing your baby cry can be enough to set milk flowing.

Almost immediately after birth a hormone, prolactin, triggers milk production in your breasts, but this milk remains stored within the sacs or alveoli in the breast until a demand for it – whether sucking on the nipple, a cry of hunger or simply touching the nipples – sends a message to the brain which releases another hormone, oxytocin. This causes the milk to flow along the milk ducts to the nipple and is known as the 'let-down reflex'.

If the milk is not called upon it will accumulate in the milk sacs, causing swelling, tenderness and what is known as engorgement, and then milk production will stop.

It is quite common, particularly to begin with, for this second stage, the let-down reflex, not to work very well. Anxiety, illness or exhaustion, the baby not suckling properly, can all interfere with this chain of reactions. And if the milk is not being used fully, less will be produced, until you have a self-fulfilling prophecy. The converse is also true: suckling more often increases milk production and prolongs lactation.

■ 'anchoring' on to the nipple. Hold your baby in towards you so there is no need to turn his or her head and check that your whole nipple and as much areola as possible is in the mouth. A baby attached to just a nipple is going to clamp on painfully and suck less efficiently.

### Relaxation

Tension doesn't help breastfeeding at all. Ask your partner to give you a massage for about 15 minutes at least once a week (see page 66). It helps to alleviate tiredness and enhances your mood as well as releasing the neck tension brought on by carrying or holding a baby, which can cause a lot of shoulder and arm pain.

### Nutrition

Through tiredness or concern about feeling fat, many women eat too little in the weeks after giving birth. Ensure you are not missing out on sufficient good-quality food – see Looking After Yourself, below.

Yam, mustard, caviar, rhubarb, grapes and soya milk are good for breast milk.

Don't forget that, because you are manufacturing the milk, something of what you eat and drink is going to be passed on to your baby. The following can have an adverse effect:

◆ over-the-counter drugs (check with your doctor and pharmacist, and read the fine print on packaging)
◆ alcohol
◆ coffee
◆ hot chillies
◆ yeast products (which can cause thrush, nappy rash, bloating, abdominal cramps or eczema)
◆ citrus fruit or vinegary foods (may cause excess acidity)
◆ excess salt
◆ excess sugar (may cause hyperactivity).

## A SPICE DRINK TO AID MILK FLOW

Boil 1 teaspoon each of aniseed, caraway seeds (ajwain) and black cumin seeds (*Nigella sativa*) in 2 litres of water for 10 minutes. Cool and add 2 tablespoons of honey. Drink this at intervals throughout the day.

In addition, be wary of canned products, which often contain surprisingly high amounts of sugar, salt or acid.

### EXPRESSING MILK

You can provide breast milk for your baby even when you are not around by expressing it from your breasts into a sterile feeding bottle. The milk can then be kept in the fridge and warmed for the next feed. This is a very useful way of allowing someone else to feed your baby and give you a rest, or to provide your own milk if your baby is in hospital because of premature delivery or ill-health.

Expressing milk can either be done by hand or with the help of a pump (both hand-operated and electrical versions are available). A good time to express milk is while your baby is feeding from one breast, as this will stimulate both breasts to release milk, and you can simultaneously bottle milk from the other breast.

Some pumps are simpler to use than others, and some women get the hang of their use more easily than others, so make sure you get good instruction from someone such as a neo-natal nurse or health visitor, and don't hesitate to ask for further help if you need it.

## Treat the mother, cure the baby

While walking with a friend of mine and her three-month-old baby girl, she told me that her daughter suffered from abdominal cramps, even though she was breastfeeding and encouraging her to burp by patting her back after almost every feed. The little girl also had bad nappy rash.

I asked to look at my friend's tongue and was not surprised to find it had a thick greying coat at the back. This told me she had candida in the gut. I discovered that she ate a yeast-based spread every day and lots of bread. I asked her to give those up and to avoid other yeasty foods. I also gave her kadu (black hellebore) tea to drink. The baby continued to have just milk, but within days her cramps had stopped and the nappy rash cleared up. A good example of how a mother's diet affects her baby's health via breast milk.

## HOW LONG TO BREASTFEED FOR?

The duration of breastfeeding has always been a debated subject. In my opinion, if the quality and quantity of milk is good and if time permits, then breastfeeding for the whole of the first year is ideal. Gradually, the milk will be supplemented by additional sustenance (see table).

## Feeding your baby

### 0 to 3 months
### milk only

Do not substitute with water even if the baby is thirsty

### 3 to 6 months
### milk + water

If the quantity of your milk reduces, start introducing solids earlier. By introducing solids, you will be relieved from night-time feeds and you will be able to sleep

### 6 months to 1 year
### at least 6 feeds a day
### + solids

Begin with soups, rice, puréed vegetables

# Mastitis and breast abscesses

If a milk duct becomes blocked, congestion builds up and your breast can become reddened and painful (mastitis). You may notice a hardening or swelling and develop a temperature. A nursing baby can also damage the skin of the areola and nipple and if bacteria enter, they thrive on the rich milk, causing infection and an abscess.

If a blockage cannot be cleared by massaging the area, or if the problem is an infection, you will have to cease breastfeeding from the affected breast until the problem is sorted out. If there is an abscess the pus has to be drained, and you may be prescribed antibiotics.

## PREVENTIVE MEASURES

Any infection is harder to fight off if you are run down due to insomnia and breastfeeding.

● When you are nursing, make sure you have vitamins and mineral supplements regularly.

● If you are exhausted (staying up all night due to frequent nursing, or if the baby is ill) make sure you have a massage once a week. Ask someone to help you so that you can have a bit of sleep during the day. Walk the baby in the park and get some fresh air. Child care is demanding and stressful, and your partner or family should get involved.

● Maintain breast hygiene and personal hygiene. Bathe regularly, washing your breasts, particularly the nipple area, with antiseptic soap wash (rinsing thoroughly with water afterwards so the baby doesn't suck it in).

# Looking after yourself Although the health of your baby is clearly the priority, do not neglect your own health and well-being.

## Nutrition

Recuperating from the birth, producing high-quality milk and reviving your energy all require a highly nutritious diet that is easy on your digestive system. Follow the general principles of the Lifestyle Programme, avoiding yeast, coffee, alcohol, citric fruits, spicy food, canned products and deep-fried food.

Eat plenty of protein and fresh fruit and vegetables, but don't cut out carbohydrates and fats: this is not the time to go on a restrictive diet. (If you are worried about your weight, see page 191). The following can help:

- the home-made chicken soup recommended on page 65; have a bowlful once a day for the first couple of weeks after the birth.
- eggs, especially when soft-boiled, are a good source of protein.
- fish roe – caviar is a traditional remedy for improving breast milk, but is expensive and over-salty; stir-fry fish roe such as cod or herring, with chopped spring onions, grated ginger, garlic and cherry tomatoes.
- avocado, cherries, apples, yam, sweet potato, bananas, pomegranate, liver and lean game, butter and ghee, honey, cottage or feta cheese; these help to nourish the body and also help milk production.
- juiced carrot, apple, celery, ginger and mint leaves.
- sweet-lime juice; this orange-like fruit with a distinct sweet-sour-bitter taste is recommended for low energy and during recuperation from illness.
- Drink plenty of fluids, including water; or carrot and apple juice, grape juice, pomegranate juice, watermelon juice and mint tea.

## AN AID TO HEALING

Boil 1 teaspoon of aniseed, a thumb-sized piece of root ginger, 5 roughly crushed cloves and 1 teaspoon of thyme or caraway seeds in 1 litre of water for 5–10 minutes. Cool and add honey. Drink this water every two hours for the first couple of days after the birth. It helps relieve any pain or discomfort, hastens recuperation and also improves secretion of breast milk.

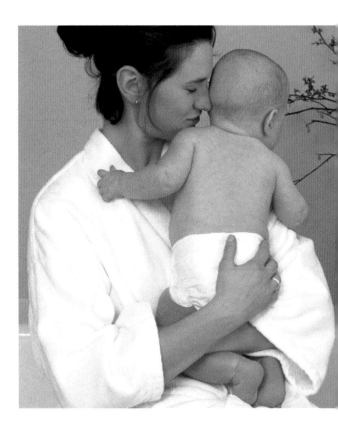

## Stay relaxed

Feeding and caring for a new baby, even with plenty of support, is a strenuous job. Being tense, worried and over-tired only makes it tougher.

- Rest as much as possible. Try and sleep when the baby does, at least twice a day.
- Don't feel shy about asking for help from family and friends with domestic matters, so that your baby can continue to be your number one priority.
- Ask your partner or a friend to massage your neck and shoulders twice a week for ten minutes or so. This helps to relieve the fatigue and restores energy. A good massage can sometimes compensate for some of the lost sleep.
- Yoga is an excellent relaxant – just 15 minutes will make all the difference. Start off with a few cycles of breathing, a few asanas for the neck and back, such as the Cobra and Semi-Bridge, and conclude with the Corpse pose (see page 157).
- Once the baby reaches two months or so, go and get some fresh air in the park. It will help both of you to feel refreshed and will encourage the baby to sleep well.

## SLEEPING ARRANGEMENTS

Having your baby beside you at night or even in bed with you may seem more convenient for night feeds, but that is one habit it is better not to form, as it will make it much more difficult to get your baby accustomed to a cot later. When, soon, your baby requires fewer feeds, sleeping separately will mean fewer disturbed nights, and your baby, too, will sleep better.

## Establishing a happy family

Building a happy, relaxed relationship with your baby will make life a lot easier later on, so don't feel guilty about taking it as easy as you can in these early days. It is important, however, that the rest of the family do not feel they have been relegated to second place.

Talk things through with them beforehand, plan special treats for all the family once the baby has arrived (even if you can't actively participate). Allow them to get involved in all aspects of caring for the new baby – there are bonds to be forged in every direction.

### SEX AFTER CHILDBIRTH

Few women feel like full sexual intercourse soon after delivery of a baby. Medically, you will usually be given the all-clear to resume sexual activities about six to eight weeks after your baby is born, but you should not worry if you feel this is still too soon. Lovemaking is more than a physical exercise, and a different sense of self, new feelings about your body, especially your breasts and vagina, lack of arousal and general fatigue all play as much a part as any remaining soreness or fear of injury.

It is important that you and your partner discuss, and keep discussing, how you both feel (he may also be confused about his changed perception of sexual and non-sexual aspects of you, especially if he was there at the actual birth). Neither of you should feel that, if you don't feel up to penetrative intercourse, there should be no intimacy. Begin to reintroduce yourselves to each other slowly, and at your own pace find all the many different ways of showing affection to each other until you regain full confidence.

# Recovering Pregnancy and childbirth have profound physical effects on the body, and you should not try to rush your recovery.

## HEALING TEARS (EPISIOTOMY; LABIAL TEARS)

A slight tearing of the perineal area (between the vagina and anus), or a small cut (episiotomy) is not uncommon during the birth. Bruising in this area is also common. To help this heal quickly, arnica 30 in tablet or drop form taken three times a day for three days is beneficial.

## HAEMORRHOIDS

Haemorrhoids (piles) can be an annoying after-effect of all the strenuous pushing of labour and delivery. Provided you do not let yourself get constipated they should shrink quite quickly, but see page 162 for help to ease them and encourage their disappearance.

## AFTER A CAESAREAN

As explained in the chapter on Pregnancy, a Caesarean section is not an easy option for childbirth, and you will probably be in hospital longer than after a vaginal birth. Once home, you will discover that almost everything you do involves your abdominal muscles, so take seriously the advice you will receive on minimizing strain but doing regular postnatal exercises. You may find holding your baby on your lap or up to your breast uncomfortable, so experiment with different methods of cushioning and support.

## REGAINING MUSCLE TONE

After delivery, the muscles and ligaments of the abdomen will be tender after having worked so hard, and lax after having been relieved of their burden. Apply arnica cream or a massage oil for backs to the abdominal muscles, particularly above the pubic bone. Apply gently, as the womb is still sensitive and there is always some residual bleeding.

Once there is no threat of further bleeding, begin massaging your abdomen with pure sweet almond oil, kneading gently with your thumbs and fingers. This will tone up the skin and help prevent the formation of stretch marks. Leave the oil to be absorbed overnight.

Try to breastfeed sitting up rather than lying on your side, especially after a meal. The abdominal wall is loose and a full stomach or intestines pressing against it may cause the central ligaments in front to stretch, and may result in a permanent bulge or herniation. You will later find your tummy beginning to bulge when you stand up, giving the false impression that you have put on weight.

From about three or four weeks after delivery you can begin to knead your lower abdomen more vigorously, using an oil formulated for cellulite (see page 292). This will help prevent the formation of that problematic 'mini-bulge' below the navel.

## LOSING EXCESS WEIGHT

A great many new mothers worry quite unnecessarily about 'all the extra weight' they have put on while pregnant that doesn't miraculously disappear as soon as the baby is born.

It is normal to put weight on during pregnancy and you will naturally lose it again. Breastfeeding is a great help here, as it helps you to regain your figure faster and more easily than if you resort early on to bottle-feeding.

Once you are home and established into a routine, you should also take into account the changed pattern of your life. Because you probably feel exhausted by the end of the day, you may feel you have done a lot but, if you stop to think, you will probably find that you are much less physically active than you used to be. Also, many women find themselves at home all day for the first time in years and, without realizing it, fill odd moments with snacks and spend a lot of time sitting down.

The chapter on Weight Control includes a lot of advice on different types of weight loss but if you didn't have a weight problem before you were pregnant, the following simple guidelines should prevent weight gain from becoming a problem.

### Diet

■ Reduce your carbohydrate intake by half. Have porridge or soda/rye bread for breakfast, and then a portion of e.g. pasta, rice, potatoes, quinoa, couscous or corn on the cob for either for lunch or dinner, but make up your third meal with just protein and vegetables.

■ Avoid excess fats. Choose lean cuts of meat, eat more fish and avoid too many heavy fats such as cream (use low-fat yoghurt instead) and butter.

■ Put a curb on snacking, and substitute fresh or dried fruit for bread or creamy, sugary nibbles. Avoid late-night snacks altogether.

### Exercise

Going to the gym or for a swim may either not be possible with a newborn reliant on you every moment or involve a disproportionate amount of preparation, and even a walk in the park can seem like too much effort. Your natural level of activity will change once your baby begins to crawl and explore, but in these first months you should ensure that you do not slip into a completely sedentary lifestyle.

■ Find a form of exercise that you can do at home in these early months. Choose something that you can do with little preparation and that you enjoy.

■ Exercise videos or DVDs can be a great help. Working with light weights, dancing and ashtanga yoga will all build up a sweat, increase your fitness and improve your shape.

■ As your baby's daily pattern becomes a little more predictable (although it will keep changing), suggest getting together with other mothers in the same situation.

If you were overweight, or found it difficult to maintain a sensible weight, before you were pregnant, you may find the excess weight more difficult to lose, especially if a hormonal imbalance is at the root of the problem. On pages 240–1 is a special feature on overcoming hormonal weight gain, but you should not go on a severely restrictive diet while you are still breastfeeding (or at any time, in fact). The steps described above, although you may notice the effect less, will still be helpful in preventing weight gain getting out of hand.

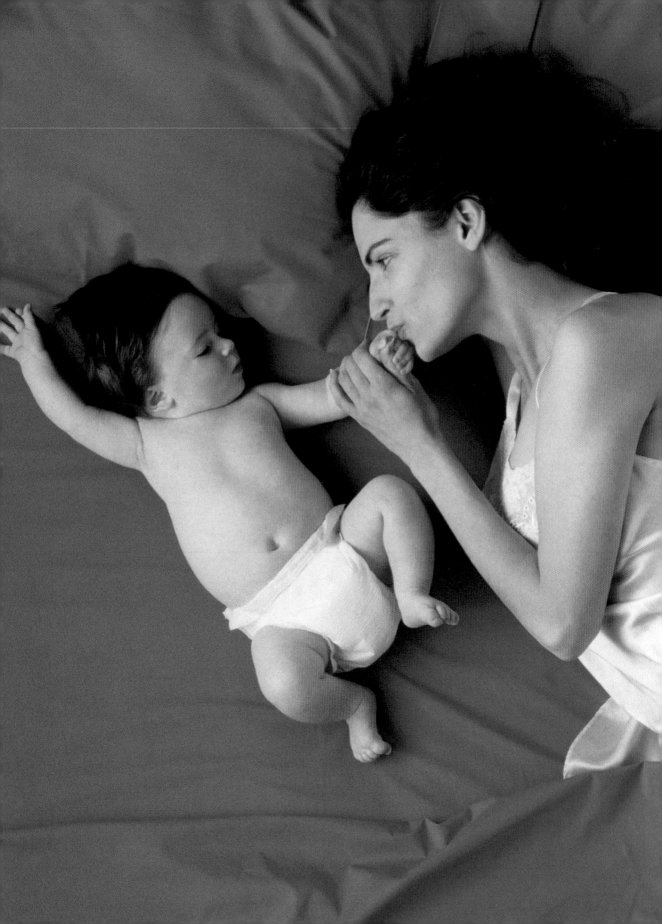

# Postnatal depression

Many mothers go through a period of despondency soon after their baby is born. This might be a lowering of the spirits that dissipates after a couple of weeks (the baby blues) or a truly depressive state that can be damaging. There are several reasons for this:

- After the surge of hormones during pregnancy, excitement about the new baby and general feeling of triumph, it is not surprising if there is a flat, let-down feeling after the euphoria wears off.

- Lack of sleep and feeling cooped up indoors with the baby (especially in winter when the days are shorter and gloomy) take their toll, perhaps exacerbated by heavy blood loss, low blood pressure or anaemia and other nutritional deficiencies (magnesium, zinc, calcium).

- Other people can make things worse. During pregnancy, a woman gets used to being fêted and cosseted, but once the baby is born much affection and attention is transferred to the new arrival. The mother's needs can be overlooked. She may be disturbed by feelings of jealousy and guilt. Such feelings can precipitate a downward spiral of resentment and lack of self-worth.

If you can't sleep well, feel low, don't want to meet people, feel like crying, want to give up everything or doubt yourself, you need help. Don't tell yourself that it's just a passing phase that every mother goes through, or that you'll be making a fuss over nothing. It might pass on its own after a month or two, but it might linger on.

Deal with it sooner rather than later. Don't try to cope on your own and don't deny that something has to be done. Your relationship with your family and the bonding with your baby may be badly affected at this crucial point.

Swallow any feelings of inadequacy, or shame, or embarrassment, and talk to someone. This might be your partner, your parents, sister, a close friend or a medical professional. Ask them to guide you through this.

*A few practical ideas:*

- Nutrition boosts mental strength as well as physical energy. Make sure your diet is highly nutritious and you are not lacking any nutrients. Common ones are protein and iron: eating spinach, liver, red meat, cherries and other good sources of iron will help correct any low blood pressure or anaemia. Drink a glass of fresh carrot, apple, ginger, celery and fresh mint juice. It will provide you with vitamins, minerals and enzymes that your body needs. Avoid the big baddies (coffee, alcohol, excess yeast and acidity) as described in the Lifestyle Programme.
- Massage and exercise are mood enhancers. Yoga can be done at home easily; it helps you to breathe and calms your mind and body. Dancing or exercise videos are also very helpful.
- This is a time to call on close family and friends. They could help you with child care, or just be with you and listen to you. Feeling you are not on your own is helpful.
- Seek professional guidance. Consult a psycho-therapist or visit an Integrated Medical Clinic.
- Resort to antidepressants only in extreme cases while you are breastfeeding.

Coping with a new baby is an art. I have just given you some essential information based on what I have learnt and observed over the years. Traditional knowledge is very important. New diseases develop and medical breakthroughs are made, but women were always pregnant and babies were always born. They knew how to deal with the situation then and their knowledge and experience is invaluable.

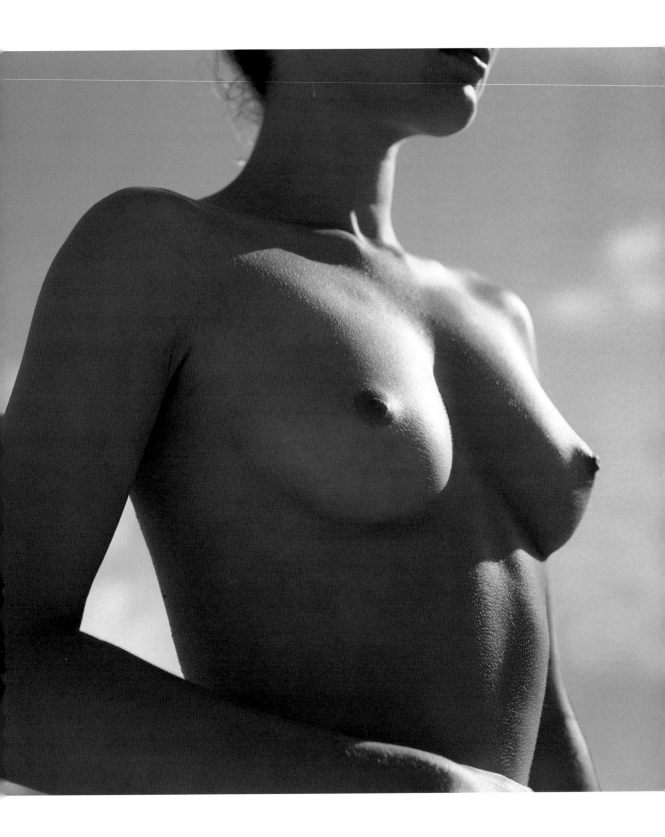

# chapter five
# breasts

Breasts are important for women in many ways. As is the case for any mammal, their practical function is to produce milk to suckle a baby, but they also play a sexual role and, being a defining female feature, their size, shape and tone are inextricably linked with how a woman feels about herself.

As a result, cosmetic surgery procedures to enhance or reduce the breasts have become more common. It is an interesting point that in societies where breasts are not usually covered, neither men nor women seem to focus on them in the way that we do in the West.

# Anatomy
Breasts consist of fat, glandular tissue, fibrous tissue, and ducts or tubes for channelling milk. It is the amount and distribution of fat that gives them their rounded contours and dictates their size.

Breasts change throughout your life. They are one of the first signs of puberty and, triggered by various hormones, start to develop before menstruation begins. The nipple and areola also change in shape, size and colour at this time, and the nipples become more sensitive to touch. Breasts will vary with your age and weight (except when you are pregnant or breastfeeding, your breasts are around 80 per cent fat), and also fluctuate slightly in size and sensitivity in the course of the menstrual cycle (see Tenderness, below).

During pregnancy, in response to progesterone, they change markedly. The nipples and areola darken and, by the later stages of pregnancy, the fatty tissue is almost completely replaced by glandular tissue. After the baby is born, under the influence of prolactin, a hormone from the pituitary gland, breasts begin to secrete milk. When nursing stops, breast tissue returns to its normal state, with an increase in fat and a decrease in glandular tissue.

After the menopause, breasts go through a further change in size and shape, losing fatty tissue and firmness (see page 306).

## Beyond the functional

Of all her features it is a woman's breasts that proclaim her femininity and in the very elderly they remain a distinguishing feature when in many other respects men and women outwardly have grown to resemble one another.

Breasts are highly sensual organs and a nipple with its surrounding areola is a powerful erogenous zone. Their sensitivity gives women pleasure and plays an important role in sexual arousal. And men are attracted to breasts, like no other mammal. Many women are reluctant to breastfeed for long as they are (wrongly) concerned about losing shapeliness and therefore reducing their attraction to men. This role in sexual attraction has led to a major industry in all sorts of cosmetic surgery and implants to enhance or reduce breasts to create 'the perfect bosom'.

However, breasts can also be a subject of embarrassment or discomfort. Many young girls are extremely shy about their burgeoning breasts, especially if they are larger or appear earlier than those of their peers. Usually this initial embarrassment soon disappears, but for some women their breasts become the focus of near-phobic concerns.

The 'normal' range for breasts is extremely varied, but the sheer weight of a very over-sized bust can cause backache and muscular strain around the shoulders and neck, as well as threatening self-confidence – not every woman can adopt an 'if you've got it, flaunt it' attitude. Such women may look enviously at flat-chested women, but having very small breasts can also be a burden. See also Premature and Delayed Puberty (page 102).

BELOW: *Unaesthetic though it sounds, milk ducts are modified sweat glands. Like all glands, they have a rich network of blood vessels. In addition, they have a network of lymphatic vessels. Within each breast are 12–20 conical lobes, with their bases near the chest wall. These taper at the top and open into the areola or nipple. Each lobe contains a central duct into which many smaller ones drain. Each major duct forms a pouch as it narrows down to reach the areola or nipple. This pouch helps the milk to drain when a baby suckles as it is siphoned out of the deeper tissue.*

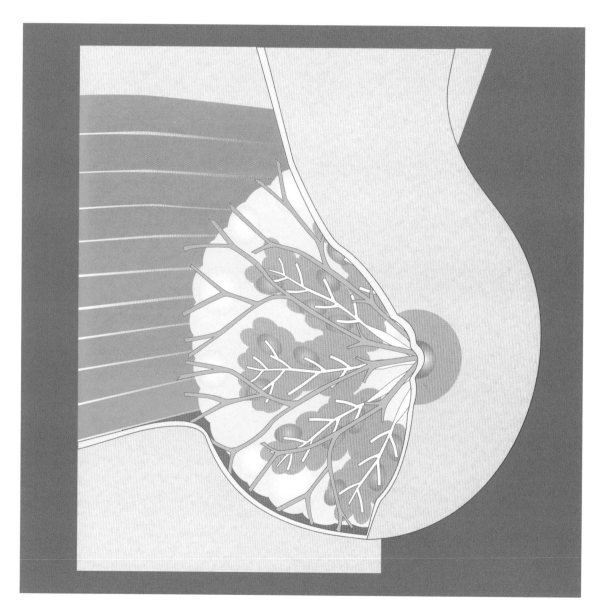

# BREAST CHECKS

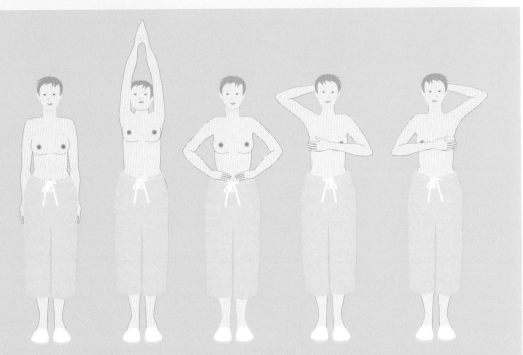

All women over the age of 20 should examine their breasts once a month. The ideal time is a few days after your period ends, as your breasts are not then swollen or tender as they may be before and during your period. Post-menopausally, do your breast examination on a fixed date every month.

Stand in front of a mirror and check your breasts visually with your arms in three different positions:

◆ by your sides.
◆ raised above your head. Press the palms of your hands against each other to flex the pectoral muscles under your breast.
◆ with elbows out and hands pressed firmly on your hips.

Can you see any signs of misshaping or unusual contours? Do they look any different from last month? Is there any discharge from around the nipples? Is there any skin rash or eczema around the nipples? (See page 203.)

Next, palpate each breast in turn. This means gently but firmly prodding your breasts with the flats of your fingertips. You may find this easier to do lying down, especially if you have large breasts. Use the left hand for the right breast and vice versa and work in concentric circles, starting from the outside and ending up near the nipple. Press the nipples gently to see if there is any discharge. What you are feeling for is any lump that has not been there before.

Finish by checking for any small, firm lumps in your armpit or up towards your neck. You have a concentration of lymph nodes here that can be affected by tumorous growths (see box, page 203).

If you see or feel anything unusual or different, go and see your GP without delay. You will probably discover that a lump is benign (see below), but the earlier the detection of anything malignant, the better the chances of successful treatment.

## Tenderness

Breasts can be become tender for a number of reasons. A young girl's growing breasts are naturally sensitive as they develop, and many women find their breasts become more tender in the pre-menstrual phase each month. This is because the glandular cells enlarge and the ducts widen, causing the breast size and firmness to increase, just as it does during pregnancy. This symptom of premenstrual syndrome (PMS) is nothing to worry about, but can be a problem when even the slightest touch by underclothing or movement causes pain, and your sleep is interrupted.

Women with hardened breast tissue (see below) find that hormonal swelling of the breasts, due to the action of progesterone, makes them tender. Sometimes the pain is very localized, usually at the site of the hardening.

For alleviating painful tenderness, see treatment under Fibrocystic Change, below.

## Nipple discharge

A discharge from the nipple or surrounding areola can be either milky or watery. Any discharge should be investigated, but a milky discharge is usually due to over-production of the hormone prolactin, which stimulates milk production. Certain drugs and contraceptive pills can sometimes cause this. It is usually more prominent before a period and disappears once the period begins.

### Treatment

The following can all help excess milk production:

◆ going on a low-protein diet for a couple of months
◆ neck and shoulder massage to improve pituitary function (prolactin stimulation comes from the pituitary)
◆ vigorous exercise.

### A SOOTHING POULTICE

A hot salt poultice can help relieve all forms of breast tenderness. Heat salt in a pan and pour into a handkerchief or square of cloth (wrap this in a second cloth if the poultice is too hot to bear). Apply it to warm the area that hurts.

*Supplements:*

◆ zinc: 15mg in tablets for a couple of months is helpful in hormone regulation
◆ there are also homeopathic remedies that can help to regulate milky secretions (consult a qualified homeopath).

For breast abscesses and mastitis, see Breastfeeding (page 187).

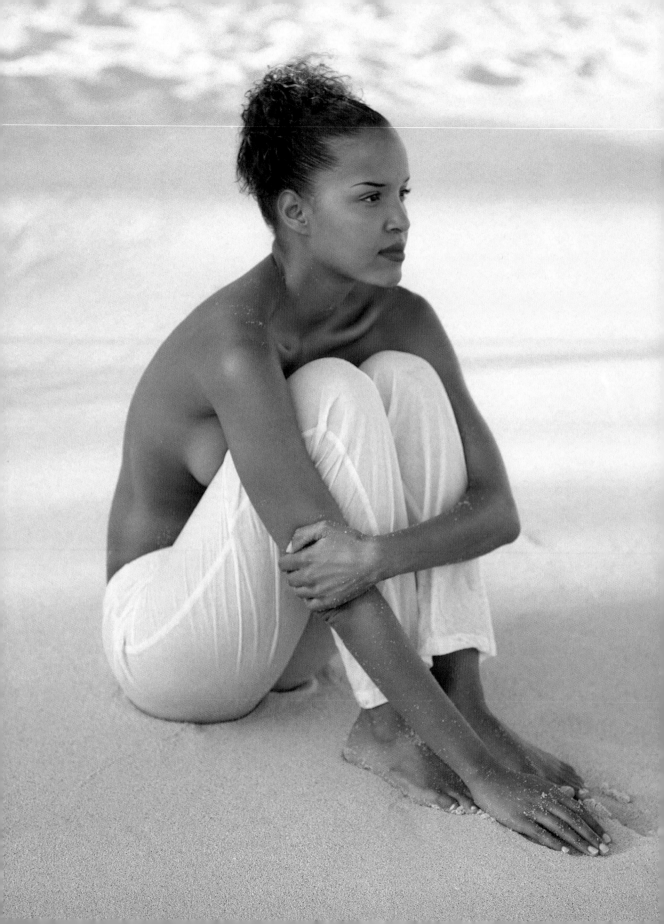

# Lumps  Self-examination is vital (see page 198), and if you find a lump you should not panic, but do seek medical advice.

It is very natural to be horrified by any lump in your breast. Whatever your age, whatever the nature of the lump, you will probably feel that a mammogram and biopsy are the very least that should be done, and straight away. If your doctor shows signs of doubt, or seems less concerned, this may add to the worry rather than be reassuring.

But most lumps are not cancerous. They should always be checked out, but it is also important for your peace of mind that you don't continue to worry unduly about a lump that has been ascertained is benign – insisting on frequent investigations 'to see if anything's changed' is not usually a sensible course.

## Fibrocystic change

Although sometimes referred to as fibrocystic disease, this is not a disease but a condition, and a common one. Fibrocystic lumps (there are often several, and commonly occur in both breasts) are often painful and tender, especially just before periods. Sometimes a discharge comes out of the nipples. They occur usually between the ages of 30 and 50 years and do not appear after menopause, and so are connected to the hormonal cycle.

So if you have several firm lumps appearing and disappearing and getting smaller as well as bigger, and if the pain or tenderness fluctuates according to the time of the month, you will almost certainly be told that fibrocystic changes are responsible. They may be worrying and uncomfortable at times, but they are benign.

**Treatment to relieve the tenderness**
Controlling the intake of certain foods and beverages can relieve the pain and tenderness to a certain extent. Avoid:

- coffee, chocolates
- excess salt
- alcohol
- spicy food
- citrus fruits
- pineapple
- mango
- yeast products
- canned products.

It is also helpful to drink a herbal tea that reduces water retention (see page 235) for a week before your periods.

Massage can soften lumps. Use cocoa butter and massage your breast before the tenderness grows (from mid-cycle to about seven days before your period).

Tenderness is made worse if your breasts move around freely, so although it may be uncomfortable, wearing a firm, supportive bra will help lessen the pain.

## Fibroadenoma

This is a common, benign hardening of the glandular tissue, more common in young women. Usually it is a hard lump that can be felt and moved around but not seen as a bump and is not tender. This sort of lump is often discovered accidentally as it does not give symptoms. Although they are benign and so relatively harmless, fibroadenomas do raise some concern in patients and doctors, so they are usually surgically removed and analysed. These lumps are often caused by cysts so full of fluid they feel hard rather than squashy.

**Breast cancer** Even though the number of cases
of breast cancer diagnosed has increased
(the chance of a woman developing breast cancer
is 1 in 8), the death rate from it has declined.

This is primarily due to early detection and treatment.
Women are now much more aware of checking their
breasts regularly for early warning signs (see Breast
Checks, page 198), and routine mammograms for
women over 50 or whose chances are greater than usual
of developing beast cancer has meant that many more
women are now surviving cancer, often without having
to resort to mastectomy (breast removal).

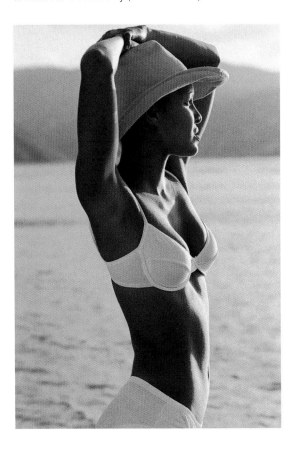

## Risk factors

While anyone is open to the possibility of developing
breast cancer, some women are at greater risk than
others. It used to be believed, for example, that only
women over 40 got breast cancer. While, sadly, even
women in their twenties can develop cancerous tumours,
you are in a low-risk group if you are under 40. So are
women who have had an artificial menopause (induced
by period-blocking drugs).

Factors that can, statistically, increase your risk of
breast cancer include:

◆ a history of breast or ovarian cancer in the family
   (particularly your mother or a sister)
◆ being over 40
◆ high oestrogen levels (contraceptive pills are no
   longer normally high-oestrogen but check HRT or
   any other hormonal treatments)
◆ starting periods early or menopause late
◆ history of benign breast disease
◆ childlessness
◆ being overweight after the menopause.

Some of these are obviously higher risk indicators than
others.

If you fall into a high-risk category it is advisable to go
for six-monthly breast examinations and ask your doctor's
advice about seeing a specialist.

# Warning signs

Around 90 per cent of breast lumps are detected by women themselves, while routine mammograms and examination by a physician frequently pick up an early sign. Not all of the following symptoms indicate cancer, but they should always be checked out straight away:

◆ appearance of any hard lump on the side of the breast, in the armpit or in the neck region
◆ breast pain
◆ nipple discharge
◆ inversion (or retraction) of nipples
◆ ulcers on the skin in the breast, neck or armpit area enlargement of one breast, resulting in abnormal lopsidedness
◆ any unusual hardness
◆ a change in shape, particularly any sort of dip or local shrinkage
◆ an area of redness or flushed skin.

In the early stage the abnormal cancerous cells form a small lump (2cm or less across) which can be moved around. Left untreated the lump grows in size and will become attached to the chest wall so that it is no longer mobile. It can also affect the skin in the form of ulcers.

# Further checks

Your doctor will arrange any suspect lump or abnormality to be investigated further, with a mammogram and/or a biopsy. A mammogram, which is a type of x-ray, gives a clearer image of a lump or abnormal tissue than manual examination can do, but a biopsy is a more accurate method of diagnosis. This involves removing a small part of the suspected tissue under local anaesthestic.

# On diagnosis

Like all cancers, breast cancer is graded according to the stage and intensity of the tumour, and treatment will depend on the results of further tests to check on the aggressiveness of its growth and its spread. Early diagnosis and treatment can make all the difference.

One important step is to establish whether the tumour cells are receptive to oestrogen or progesterone (that is, they seem to grow rapidly when the level of these hormones in blood is high: see risk factors, above). If they are, then drugs to block these hormones can often successfully contain or suppress the growth of the cells. This gives a positive prognosis.

## SIGNIFICANCE OF LYMPH NODES

Rather like the blood circulation system, the lymph network runs all over your body. It is fed by glands or nodes, and one of the areas of concentration of these is close to the breasts, clustered in and around the armpit and up towards the neck. If cancerous cells in the breast reach the lymph nodes, the worry is that the lymph system will provide the means for them to spread more rapidly to other areas of the body.

This is why, as well as any lump in a breast itself, you should be alert to the appearance of any tell-tale lumps in the area of your armpit or neck. They will be small, hard and round, and able to be moved around.

# Conventional treatments

The most suitable treatment will very much depend on what stage the cancer has reached and the prognosis. Choice of treatment will also be influenced by your age and general state of health. If you are elderly, for instance, your metabolism will be slower than a young woman's and the cancer likely to be much slower in growth, so invasive treatment could well represent a greater danger than the tumour itself.

# Surgery

This can range from a lumpectomy (removal of lump and some surrounding tissue) to a total mastectomy (removal of entire breast). If done soon after diagnosis in the early stages a lumpectomy is often very successful when combined with general health and stress management.

# Chemotherapy

There is no doubt that the various chemotherapeutic drugs used to destroy cancer cells can be very effective, and if the toxic effects on the body were not so harmful, this would be a great treatment. Common side-effects (which vary according to the mix of drugs and the individual) include nausea, fatigue, loss of appetite, hair loss and a weakened immune system.

However, there is much you can do to offset or combat the potential damage (see page 277). It is unfortunate that people in the late stages of cancer are given massive doses of chemotherapy in a bid to 'kill the cells off'. It's not that simple. Chemotherapeutic drugs drastically weaken the body, the main organs (liver and kidneys) and other tissues struggle to return to their

normal level of activity, and hence the immune system fails.

### RADIOTHERAPY

This is a form of x-ray or radioactive 'zapping' that precisely targets specific locations (including lymph nodes), burning the tissue to destroy malignant cells. It is a very useful treatment for cancerous cells that are not widespread, and as a precaution against any malignant cells not excised during surgery. It does not damage the rest of the body, but burnt tissue can act as a burden to the immune system. Your body perceives the burnt cells as 'dead' so it tries to summon up antibodies to deal with them, and also expends energy creating scar tissue. On the plus side, this stimulation of the immune system may work beneficially, like vaccination or a bout of infection does.

# Integrated medical therapy

I do not dismiss conventional treatments at all, but I do not believe they should be stand-alone answers. Integrating an appropriate form of conventional therapy (surgery and/or radiotherapy as the preferred option and less-aggressive chemotherapy as well if necessary) with a lifestyle that gives your body the strength to combat what has invaded it – both the cancer and the damaging treatments – is more likely to reach remission and possibly cure.

Unfortunately, the doses of chemotherapeutic drugs are typically calculated by body weight and not by an individual's requirement. It is worth discussing with the oncologist the possibility of a lower dose of less-toxic drugs. Some may be sympathetic, especially when they know you are making major changes in your lifestyle so that the drugs are being combined with a good diet, health-building measures, stress management and some supplements. This would be true integrated medical therapy.

## DIET

The principles behind these guidelines are simple:
◆ good nourishment
◆ easy digestion and elimination (so that your body's energy and resources are not unnecessarily diverted)
◆ weight maintenance: the illness and the worry are likely to make you lose weight, and you should keep up your reserves of energy at a time like this.

*I recommend the following:*
◆ Read and follow carefully the dietary advice in the Lifestyle Programme.
◆ Eat organic food whenever you can, and make sure it is as fresh as possible: vegetables and fruit, in particular, begin to lose their nutritional value as soon as they are picked.
◆ Raw fruits and vegetables will supply potent enzymes, and many are richer in certain vitamins and minerals than when they are cooked.
◆ Make sure you are getting sufficient protein (egg, fish, chicken), especially if you are underweight.
◆ Following the Lifestyle Programme means avoiding excess salt and sugar and fried foods. However, these all add flavour to food, and if your appetite is poor bland food won't help, even if it is easy on the digestion. Stimulate your appetite with flavoursome herbs and spices (see ideas in the chapter on Weight Control).
◆ Have regular mealtimes, and never too late in the evening. This might affect your sleep, and sleep is an important healing factor.

◆ Prevent constipation with high-fibre foods such as prunes, papaya, figs, spinach, beetroot and porridge.
◆ Keep up your fluid intake to help flush your system: drink 1½–2 litres of water every day.

## MASSAGE

Many physicians think that because massage improves blood and lymph circulation, it helps to spread the cancer, and so patients are often alarmed when massage is recommended. If that were true, then exercise would do more or less the same. It is important, though, that any massage is done by a trained massage therapist who knows about your condition. Correct massage aids the healing process (see page 66) because of the sense of well-being it brings, and this is extremely important for healing because the body and mind are then in an optimum state to function better. Feeling good motivates the body to heal itself.

## AND FOR ENERGY...

◆ A super juice: carrot, apple, root ginger, fresh mint and sprouted beans/seeds (alfalfa or wheatgerm or bean sprouts). This helps to energize the body and keep the bowel movements in order.
◆ Almonds (soaked beforehand for 24 hours) with a little honey in the morning.
◆ Ginger tea: either slices of fresh, or a spoonful of powdered, ginger added to hot water (with or without milk) with honey to taste.

## EXERCISE, RELAXATION AND MEDITATION

Hatha yoga, with its calming breathing techniques and ability to still your mind and calm your body, is exactly what you need. The pace of life is fast, the level of anxiety in society is very high, and your personal anxiety levels are probably going to be sky-high; you need an antidote. The Living Yoga through-the-day routines (see pages 76–81) are sufficient to keep your mind and body in tune with each other, but you might also like to go to a regular yoga class, or engage a teacher.

Meditation has an important role to play in the healing process too. It is a powerful way of relieving the inevitable stress, inducing a state of calm and well-being, and many people recovering from cancer have found it has brought them the strength they need through a difficult time.

No cancer therapy can be complete without incorporating relaxation techniques. There are many techniques through which you can learn to still and control your mind through relaxation, breathing and meditation.

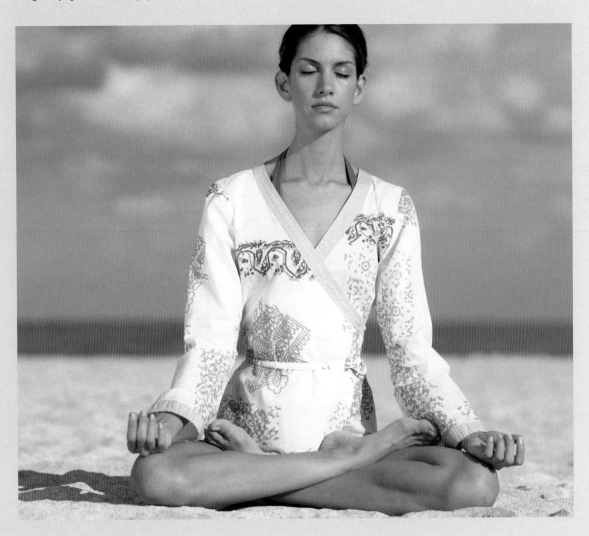

## SUPPLEMENTS

The toxic drugs used in chemotherapy give the liver and the immune system a heavy battering. The need for micro-nutrients is greater as the body tries to rectify the damage as soon as possible, but this is often hindered by a loss of appetite and an under-functioning liver. Boosting your supply of nutrients with vitamin and mineral supplements helps your body to carry out its normal functions and creates the feel-good factor so necessary for cancer therapy.

◆ To maximize your intake of nutrients it is worth considering intravenous infusions of vitamins and minerals (administered by a doctor), before and after chemotherapy. The effectiveness of this therapy is often debated, but patients do feel better for it and find that the effects of chemo- and radiotherapy are not so devastating. The supply of these nutrients helps the body to spring back more quickly to the level of well-being before the chemo- or radiotherapy treatment.

◆ Oral multivitamins and minerals can be taken in between the infusions, as a general nutritional boost.

Over the past decades, I have met many survivors of breast and other cancers who refused simply to go along the prescribed path of chemo-radiotherapy and have had amazing results. Gerson therapy, naturopathy and various herbal therapies have produced many successes. It should be stressed that many have not been successful, as with many conventional treatments.

Unorthodox treatments are generally not looked upon favourably by conventional doctors, and trials have proved difficult to conduct fairly. (A trial testing natural methods carried out in a leading London research institute ended disastrously. It appeared that only terminally ill patients were given the opportunity to try unorthodox measures,

whereas the group receiving conventional treatment consisted of patients in varying stages.)

The rate of survival in breast cancer is far better than many other forms of cancer. Many doctors have begun to recognize the power of 'other treatments' (sometimes in combination with orthodox treatments). There are many success stories and these are called 'spontaneous remissions' or 'anecdotal cases'. Whatever the term for them, the success stories are out there.

A further consideration is quality of life. It is important to make informed choices and follow the line you feel most happy with. There are times when the pursuit of extending life in any form is worse – for those around you as well as for yourself – than pursuing a high quality of life.

## FURTHER THOUGHTS

When I was a medical student in Moscow, the Head of the Department of Anatomy was doing research on the microcirculatory network of blood vessels that precedes tumour growth. She found that a network of blood vessels began to multiply rapidly (like branches of a tree) before cells began to grow on them (like leaves or buds). She felt that if there was any permanent cure for cancer, it would be to identify these areas where blood vessels begin to branch, and block them – no blood supply means no tumour growth. Today, more than 30 years later, scientists are looking for ways to do that. Breast cancer would be a primary candidate for such treatment as the area is more easily accessible than, for instance, deep in an internal organ.

*See also ... the chapter on General Disorders and Problems for more help on coping with long-term illness and recuperation from surgery.*

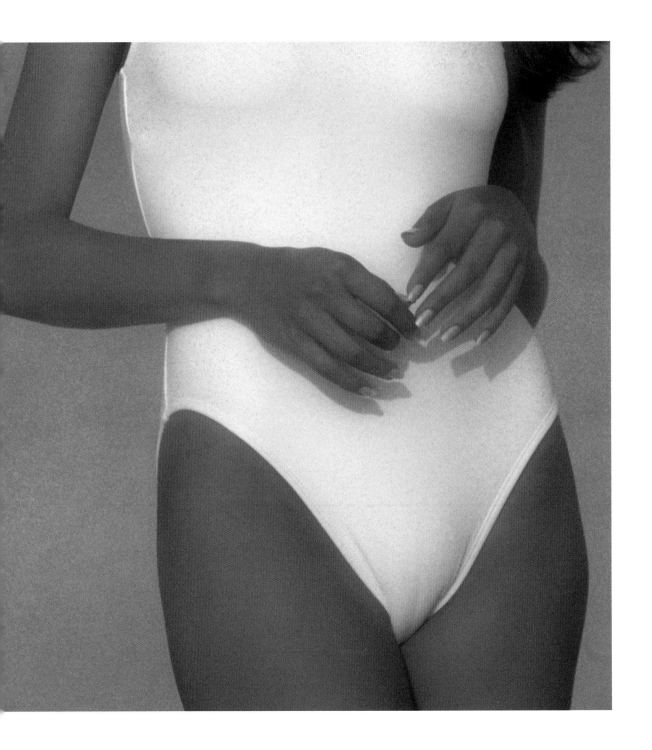

# chapter six

# vaginal and urinary health

Although the vagina and the urinary tract are not directly connected, their proximity means that trouble with one can rebound on the other. As every pregnant woman knows, for instance, a swelling uterus puts a good deal of pressure on the bladder. It is also the same set of muscles that hold both bladder and uterus in place, so a weakness here will affect both.

# An anatomical guide
Understanding the processes taking place in your vaginal and urinary systems is important for maintaining the health of these areas.

BELOW: *Urine is produced by our kidneys and passes, via the ureters, into the bladder. When this is full, the urine is released down the urethra and out of the body. To control where and when we do this the brain receives a message that our bladder needs emptying and we can, to a greater or lesser extent, use muscles to temporarily stop urine from being released. The uterus sits just above and behind the bladder and is similarly connected to the* outside world, by the vagina. The vagina is about 8cm long and lined with strong but involuntary muscles (these can only be controlled at will with specific training). The vagina is kept lubricated by secretions from the cervix, and additional lubrication during sexual stimulation is supplied by small glands (Bartholin's glands) near the vagina entrance.

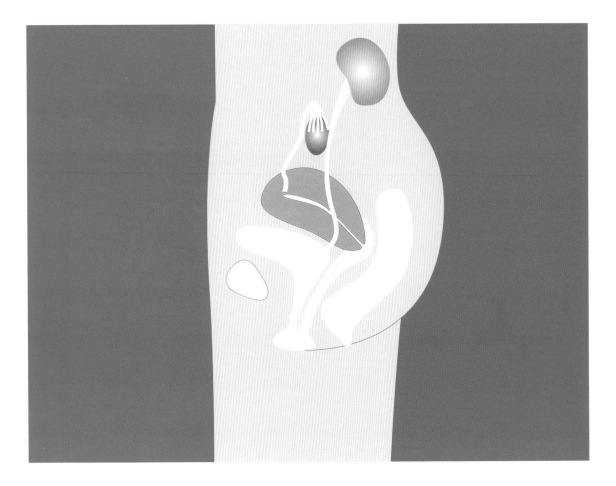

# Problems

Both the urethra and the vagina are vulnerable to irritation and infection because they connect directly with the outside world and provide the sort of warm dampness that bacteria and fungi prefer. However, they have built-in mechanisms to offset this vulnerability. The urethra is protected by urine itself, which is sterile and, provided there is a good flow, helps flush out anything unwanted, acting much like an internal douche. The vagina, at least during a woman's reproductive years, constantly sheds layers of lining to keep itself fresh, and maintains a specific pH (acid/alkaline) balance that inhibits pathogenic bacterial or fungal growth.

It is when these mechanisms go wrong that most problems occur. It is sensible to treat them as soon as possible, not only because they are irritating and highly uncomfortable, but because, left untreated, they can spread upwards and cause greater problems to other organs, such as the kidneys or ovaries.

## CYSTITIS

This is inflammation of the urinary tract, often because of an infection. It is characterized by an urgent need to pass water frequently, even when your bladder is not full, and a burning or stinging sensation while doing so. It can be accompanied by pain above the pubic region, headaches and nausea, and can develop into a low-grade fever (especially in the late afternoon), shakes and chills and general weakness and body ache. Cloudy and smelly urine should confirm the diagnosis.

Cystitis is very common (about 50 per cent of women have experienced an attack at some time), and for many women it becomes a recurrent problem. It can be kickstarted by anything that irritates your urethra, and a particular sensitivity may set it off time and again. Wearing synthetic or non-absorbent underwear, internal abrasion caused by energetic sex or an activity such as horse-riding, contact with perfumed bath oils or talc, or chlorine (in swimming pools), and oral sex can all be culprits. 'Honeymoon cystitis' is quite common, and is caused by bruising around the urethra as a result of overenthusiastic lovemaking. Even urine itself can be responsible, if it is either over-acidic or too concentrated (from drinking too few fluids).

## Pelvic floor exercises

The various organs of the lower part of the abdomen are held in place by pelvic muscles and ligaments that lie in hammock-like fashion from front to back. Keeping this support well-toned and strong helps bladder control, muscular control during sexual intercourse, and reduces the risk of prolapse (see page 217).

Exercising the pelvic floor can be done at almost any time and is discreet enough even to be done in public. Aim to do it often, about once an hour. There are several variant exercises, but you could try the following:

Push down, as if you were trying to go to the toilet, hold for 5 seconds and then pull in the opposite direction, as if you were trying to suck your rectum up into your stomach. Hold for 5 seconds. Repeat four or five times.

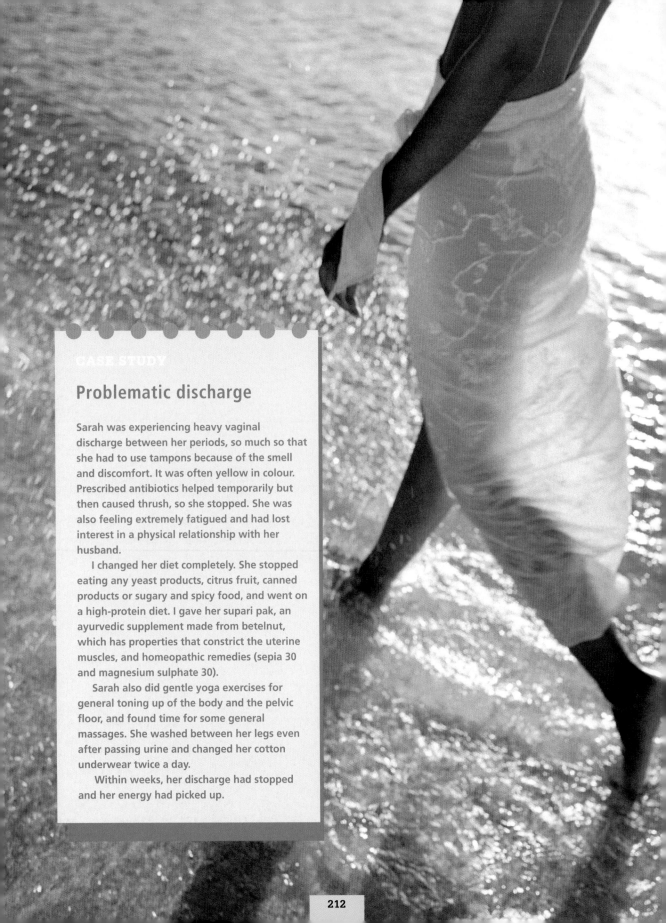

## Problematic discharge

Sarah was experiencing heavy vaginal discharge between her periods, so much so that she had to use tampons because of the smell and discomfort. It was often yellow in colour. Prescribed antibiotics helped temporarily but then caused thrush, so she stopped. She was also feeling extremely fatigued and had lost interest in a physical relationship with her husband.

I changed her diet completely. She stopped eating any yeast products, citrus fruit, canned products or sugary and spicy food, and went on a high-protein diet. I gave her supari pak, an ayurvedic supplement made from betelnut, which has properties that constrict the uterine muscles, and homeopathic remedies (sepia 30 and magnesium sulphate 30).

Sarah also did gentle yoga exercises for general toning up of the body and the pelvic floor, and found time for some general massages. She washed between her legs even after passing urine and changed her cotton underwear twice a day.

Within weeks, her discharge had stopped and her energy had picked up.

## Preventive measures

Cystitis, especially if it flares up frequently, can curtail your social life, your sex life and make everyday events such as a journey to work or school a fraught experience.

- Identify any main triggers. Some common ones are mentioned on page 211, but you may be able to trace the problem to something specific, such as a badly fitting contraceptive diaphragm or the use of a particular brand of washing powder.

- The most common cause of an infection is bacteria from faeces, so personal hygiene is an important preventive, and always wipe your bottom from front to rear to minimize contamination. Use wet tissues to wipe if you have frequent cystitis.

- Every day, drink at least 2 litres of water, or fluids recommended opposite.

- Wear only cotton underwear and avoid very tight-fitting trousers.

- Ask someone to give you a neck and shoulder massage. It relieves stress and improves blood flow to the pituitary, controller of the immune system.

Even if you have never had cystitis, take these precautions if your natural defences are weakened, either from illness or as a result of chemotherapy or radiotherapy, or if you are just run down. Cystitis is also more common in the later stages of pregnancy.

## Treatments

A urine sample will identify if an infection is present and the bacteria responsible. Usually antibiotics are prescribed, a general one at first followed by a specific one. All the symptoms of cystitis can occur without being initiated by bacteria (see Interstitial Cystitis, overleaf).

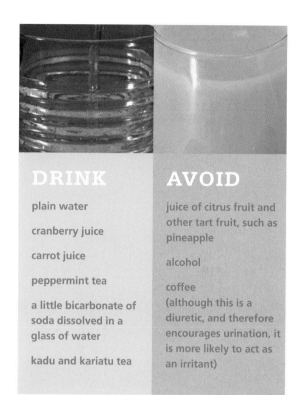

| DRINK | AVOID |
|---|---|
| plain water | juice of citrus fruit and other tart fruit, such as pineapple |
| cranberry juice | |
| carrot juice | alcohol |
| peppermint tea | coffee (although this is a diuretic, and therefore encourages urination, it is more likely to act as an irritant) |
| a little bicarbonate of soda dissolved in a glass of water | |
| kadu and kariatu tea | |

What you eat, and especially drink, will do a lot to ease the symptoms. Don't cut down on your fluid intake because urinating is painful – passing plenty of water will help the condition clear up more quickly, and the urine itself, because it is more dilute, will be less of an irritant. What you drink makes a difference. Avoid anything acidic and choose 'alkalizing' drinks instead (see box).

Avoid yeast products, chillies, ginger, garlic and canned products, as these tend to increase the burning sensation.

*Supplements:*

- shilajit, an Indian remedy made from Himalayan rock or bitumen, has many useful minerals, including magnesium and zinc. These help to alkalize the urine, reducing the burning or stinging sensation as well as improving the immune system.
- cantharis 30 is a useful homeopathic preparation: take three or four times a day at the onset of an attack.

# INTERSTITIAL CYSTITIS

Many of the symptoms of cystitis – frequent need to urinate, a burning sensation, a feeling of fullness in the bladder – can occur without there being a bacterial infection. Antibiotics are no help in these cases. How can you get a sensation of a full bladder and yet pass very little urine? What can be causing the burning pain if there is no infection?

I have noticed that most people diagnosed with this form of cystitis, called interstitial or non-specific, have a marked soreness in the tendons that join the abdominal muscles to the pubic bone.

These lower abdominal tendons can easily get inflamed or strained due to injury, excessive strain or the repetitive movements of some exercises or sports. I believe that the burning pain from the tendons gives a false impression of a full bladder and irritation inside it – the sensation does not originate in the bladder but feels as if it does.

Following this hypothesis, many of my patients have found that massaging these tendons three times a day, just as described for relief from severe period pain (see page 93), is a successful answer to the problem.

## THRUSH

About 75 per cent of women will at some time experience an attack of thrush, or vaginal candidiasis. The most common cause is *Candida albicans*, a type of fungus that thrives on the mucous lining of the throat, mouth, large intestines and vagina.

Candida is always present in the body but is usually kept under control. It gets the upper hand when its controls, such as bacteria in the gut or the body's immune system, falter. Diabetes, HIV, obesity and ME all open the way for this opportunistic fungus. Certain drugs, such as antibiotics (which kill good bacteria along with harmful ones), contraceptive pills, HRT, chemotherapy or steroids, and the chemicals used in condoms and tampons can also aggravate the situation.

Symptoms are usually a painfully itchy vulva and an excessive vaginal discharge which is white and curd-like. The itching can cause ulceration from scratching, sexual intercourse is uncomfortable and it can be painful to pass water as urine stings the inflamed vulva. Some women find it gets worse just before their period. The infection can be so recurrent that it gives the impression of being chronic.

## Treatments

Conventional medical treatment of candidiasis calls on anti-fungal drugs and steroid creams used over a period of time. If the cause can be traced to a particular contraceptive pill or drug, then, unless unavoidable, it may be necessary to stop using it.

Since an excess of Candida means that fungi and yeasts have got the upper hand in the body, avoid yeast, fungi and fermented products altogether. These include:

◆ bread, including pizza and flatbreads containing yeast
◆ yeast extract spread
◆ gravy granules
◆ beer (including lager and Guinness)
◆ wine
◆ vinegar
◆ mushrooms
◆ cheese
◆ grapes (these carry a white fungus on their skin).

Also avoid excess sugars and carbohydrates, as these are the primary food of yeasts and fungi. And do not drink anything that will make your urine more acidic (see Cystitis, page 211), as this will further irritate your labia.

*The following are all helpful:*

◆ anti-fungal products such as caprylic acid and grapefruit seed extract

◆ Kadu and Kariatu, natural ayurvedic products that help to restrict yeast, candida and fungal overgrowth

◆ a vaginal compress, made from a pad of cotton wool soaked in live yoghurt, as a calmant

◆ zinc supplement

◆ multivitamins, to boost the body's ability to fight off infection

◆ neck massage for stress relief.

## PELVIC INFLAMMATORY DISEASE (PID)

Pelvic inflammatory disease is usually a result of an infection or smaller complaint that has gone untreated and has developed into a problem that can have some serious consequences, including infertility. PID can arise from an infection such as chlamydia (see page 139) that has spread upwards from the vagina, inflammation from an intra-uterine contraceptive device, ovarian or tubular abscesses, or a complication after an abdominal operation. It can occur in several forms, one of the most common being acute salpingitis (inflammation of the Fallopian tubes).

PID can come in the form of a single attack (typically characterized by sharp abdominal pain and a temperature) or become a chronic condition. Symptoms can include:

◆ acute abdominal pain

◆ backache

◆ unusual vaginal discharge or bleeding

◆ a bout of fever accompanied by shivering

◆ pain when urinating

◆ feeling sick and losing appetite, resulting in weight loss.

**Treatment**

Antibiotics are the most common method of treatment, but if the infection does not respond, surgery may be necessary.

Adhering to the Lifestyle Programme, and supplementing your diet with multivitamins and minerals, will help improve your immune system and assist your body in combating the infection and coping with the side-effects of antibiotics, which include thrush, intestinal candidiasis (bloating, gas and lethargy), diarrhoea and occasionally a skin rash.

## A worrying irritation

A Middle Eastern lady had suffered from vaginal irritation for years, with symptoms of burning urine and an itchy and burning sensation in her vagina. Physical contact with her husband had become painful and uncomfortable. This was straining their marital relationship, and she feared that he would take another wife. She had seen several specialists who diagnosed the condition as 'non-specific vaginitis'. Antibiotics were frequently prescribed without much effect, and in fact had brought on bouts of thrush. She had also been prescribed steroid creams, without much long-term effect. At this point she came to see me in London.

Her diet explained everything: she loved lemons, oranges, pickled vegetables, chillies and tomatoes, and drank freshly squeezed lemon in hot water every morning to keep her weight under control (a myth that many adhere to). I advised her to stop eating and drinking anything acidic or sour, and gave her some ayurvedic remedies to reduce the acidity of her urine. Within a month, the problem had disappeared.

## INCONTINENCE

Incontinence is an uncomfortable and embarrassing problem that, when serious, can affect your whole quality of life. Shame, depression and the constant worry about the whereabouts of the nearest toilet can colour everything you do.

◆ Bladder control can be impaired by many things, including:
◆ age – in your 60s and 70s your muscles, like your skin, lose elasticity, and there is a general loosening of muscles in the pelvic area
◆ damage to the pubic region
◆ an over-stretched pelvic floor (from a strenuous labour)
◆ prolapse (see below)
◆ multiple sclerosis (where damage to areas of the spinal cord lead to malfunction of the nerves that control the bladder)
◆ complication resulting from an epidural injection (for pain relief in labour or for backache)
◆ nervous or psychological problems.

Temporary or occasional problems can also be caused by:
◆ diabetes, where it causes excess urine production
◆ cystitis
◆ chronic constipation, causing pressure on the bladder from distended intestines
◆ increase in abdominal pressure, from laughing, sneezing, coughing, etc.

### Treatments

A urinary tract infection or problems in the wake of childbirth are common causes of incontinence, so the first step must be to consult a urologist or a gynaecologist to find out the cause. Treatment will depend on diagnosis.

If, as is quite often the case, a contributory cause is weakness rather than permanent damage to the pelvic floor muscles, strengthening these will make a big difference. See page 211 for a simple pelvic floor exercise and the yoga pose for another helpful variation.

Your doctor may also suggest bio-feedback, which uses an electronic pressure catheter to teach you control over the muscles that close the urethra.

The following will also help ease the problem:

◆ Avoid cold water and chilled drinks, ice cubes, coffee or caffeinated drinks (which are diuretic), alcohol, excess salt, canned products, very spicy food, citrus and sour fruit.
◆ Don't limit your fluid intake, but drink only in small amounts at a time throughout the day, rather than taking large draughts all at once.
◆ Massage above the pubic bone (see page 105); this may relieve the urgency and subconscious urge to empty your bladder.
◆ Relaxation and visualization techniques are very useful.
◆ There are drugs available for extreme cases, but these can have side-effects.

## UTERINE OR VAGINAL PROLAPSE

The pelvic floor is like a basin supported at its rim by the coccyx (tail bone) and lower parts of the pelvic bone. This basin is what supports the weight of all the organs in the pelvis. Weakness in the muscles or ligaments of this basin, or increased pressure on it, can cause an area to herniate, which means that, without support, an organ such as the uterus can drop, or prolapse. There can be vaginal, urethral or rectal prolapses.

*Uterine prolapse usually happens due to:*
◆ the strain of multiple births
◆ obesity and chronic severe coughing, probably from asthma or bronchitis
◆ local conditions such as fluid retention in the abdomen, fibroids or other tumours that have grown large
◆ excessive high-impact exercises, especially if you have fibroids or a tumour, or heavy weightlifting over a period of time
◆ weakness of muscles and ligaments of the pelvic floor.

## Asana to exercise the pelvic floor

Stand erect with feet hip-distance apart. Breathe in and divert all your attention to your pelvic floor, letting it go and visualizing it bulging downwards. Breathe out and at the same time suck your pelvic floor up as high as it will go. Hold for a count of five each time. This requires a bit of practice, but once perfected it can help to strengthen the pelvic floor muscles. Do this two or three times a day, preferably on an empty stomach.

*Prolapses vary greatly in their degree.*
◆ Mild prolapse is felt as a firm mass in the vagina.
◆ With moderate prolapse, the cervix has descended to the lower part of the vagina. At this stage, it may feel like sitting on a ball or something is falling out. There may be a feeling of heaviness in the area, low backache and abdominal pulling and some incontinence of urine.
◆ In severe prolapse, the cervix appears outside the vagina, inverting the vaginal wall. Being exposed to the atmosphere causes the extrusion to become dry, often bleeding and prone to forming ulcers. There may be unpleasant discharge or bleeding. Pressure on the bladder will affect urination (urinary tract infection is a common complication) and there may be constipation or haemorrhoids, or defecation may be painful due to pressure on the colon.

### Treatments

Prolapse doesn't usually happen suddenly, and acting on early warning signs can prevent the problem progressing to the advanced stages. Pelvic floor exercises (see page 211) can help, but only in the initial stage or if the prolapse is mild. These exercises are also an important preventive measure.

Post-menopausally, oestrogen therapy (HRT) helps maintain the tone of the pelvic floor.

A vaginal pessary can used to prevent a mild prolapse from getting worse.

With more serious degrees of prolapse, surgery may be the only option (see Hysterectomy, page 112).

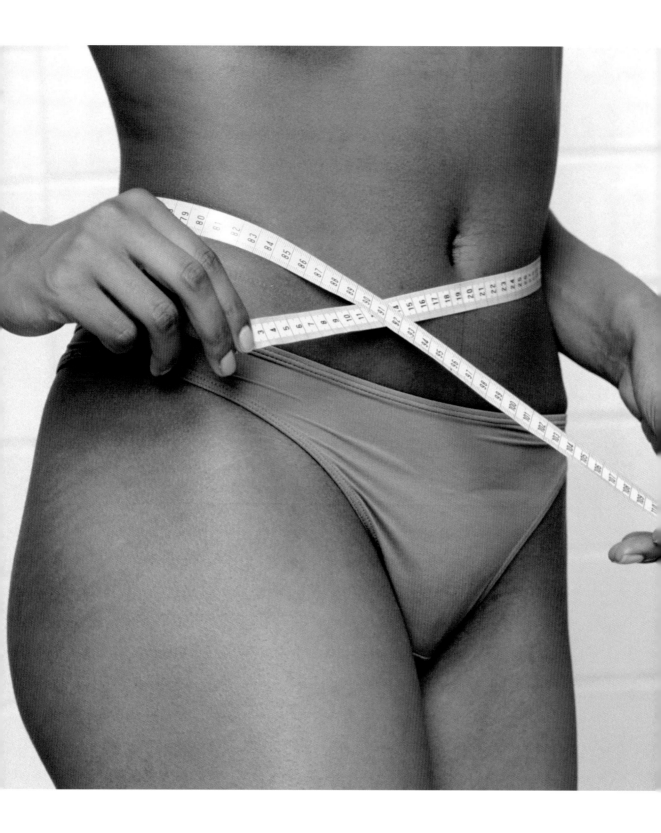

# chapter seven

# weight control

Weight is a big issue for both men and women, but is of greater concern to women. Not only do women worry more about it, both from the point of view of health and looks, but often they take on the worry of the whole family's weight, whether it's a partner's paunch, a child getting insufficient exercise and inappropriate food at school or an elderly parent's growing rotundity.

Twenty years ago I would have said that there was too much concern about weight, and that there was an unhealthy obsession with trying to look like a stick-thin supermodel. But, mostly as a result of unhealthy eating and increasingly sedentary lifestyles, obesity truly is a problem, and one that is reaching epidemic proportions.

# Health and happiness Most of us want to lose weight to improve the way we look, but of bigger concern are the health problems that excess weight brings.

The best way of not having to lose weight, of course, is to avoid the problem in the first place. Following the Lifestyle Programme is an excellent guard against eating too much or eating the wrong things; the relaxation element will help you to avoid turning to food for comfort and the exercise will ensure you don't lay up unnecessary stores of fat.

Reaching and maintaining a sensible weight is a vital part of optimum health, but something that many, many women have trouble with. With so many diet guides and

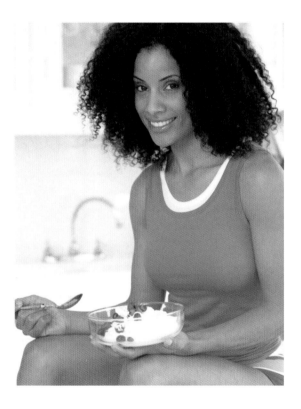

## THE PROBLEMS TOO MUCH WEIGHT CAN BRING

Being overweight affects much more than just your waistline and your ability to exert yourself without feeling sticky and exhausted. Repercussions for your health include:

◆ increased chances of a heart attack, especially once you reach the menopause
◆ strain on the joints
◆ high blood pressure and clogged arteries
◆ breathing problems, if you are very overweight
◆ fertility problems
◆ increased risk of gall stones
◆ increased risk of osteoarthritis
◆ associated psychological problems if you feel unhappy with your size.

Excess weight has also been associated with certain types of cancer, including breast, colon and endometrial cancers.

so much advice around, this may seem surprising. But time and again I hear: 'However little I eat, it never makes any difference', 'I lose weight, and then as soon as I stop dieting I put it all back on again', 'My sister's fat, my mother's fat – what chance have I got?' And in these cries of woe lie two key points:

■ not everyone is fat for the same reasons

■ the way to a healthy weight is a sensible eating plan for life, not switching from one regime to another in the hope of finding a magical quick fix.

# Overweight and infertile – and very unhappy

Geeta was 35, obese and had had no periods for two years. Her doctor told her she could never have a child because she was obese and prematurely menopausal. The same opinion from several specialists had made her extremely depressed.

She came to me initially for advice on preventing osteoporosis. However, on going through her medical history, I learned that she had had several accidents, including whiplash injuries and a broken tooth. She also suffered from headaches, food cravings, low thyroid function, dizziness, sleep disturbances and memory loss – all symptoms of poor blood supply to the subconscious brain.

I asked her to follow the Lifestyle Programme and the ultra-low fat diet for hormonal weight gain. She ate no fats, fasted once a week, took Hormone Support and Mexican yam capsules, and had neck therapy under one of my assistants at the clinic. She also began walking regularly and going to the gym twice a week.

After four months, she had her first period – I remember her excitement when she called up to share the news. She had lost nearly 13kg and felt great. Her periods became regular and a year later she conceived and had a healthy baby. Her worry and tensions in the family were over.

The neck treatments helped the pituitary, and so the thyroid and ovaries, to function better. The diet and exercise helped her lose weight and build self-confidence. In all, her body began to work as it should.

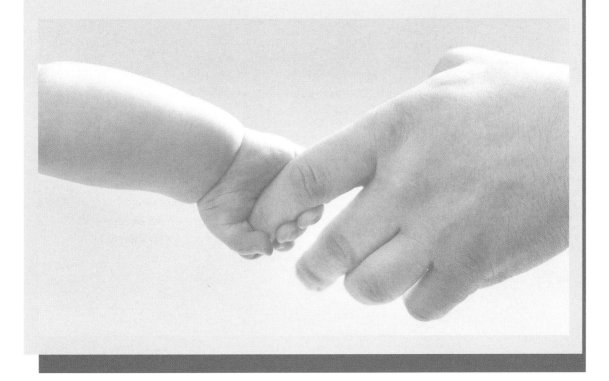

# Weight gain: the reasons Excess weight can have just one cause, but quite often there are a number, working together to exacerbate and complicate things.

## OVEREATING OR EATING THE WRONG THINGS

This, as you might expect, is the most common reason for weight gain. Sometimes it is sheer greed, but often it involves eating more than you need because you always have, and don't recognize you are overeating, or eating foods that you don't realize are contributing to your problem, or using food as a psychological prop rather than a fuel. Eating too much often goes hand in hand with:

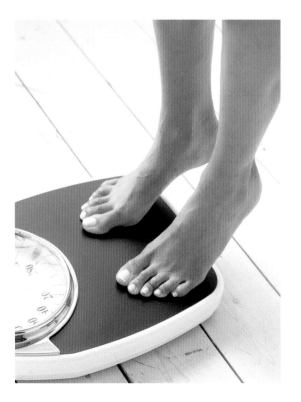

## Too little exercise

What you eat is converted into energy, either for your body to use straight away or to store for later use. Even basic functions, such as thinking, or your heart pumping, call on energy reserves but, as I shall explain in a little more detail later, if we expend less energy than we consume, our bodies store it in the form of fat.

## Hormones

Although men can be beset by hormonal problems that cause weight increase, this is a far more common problem for women. A hormonal imbalance can result in a variety of weight-related problems, including fluid retention, an unregulated appetite centre and, an often misunderstood symptom, the accumulation of cellulite, or white fat (see box, page 240).

## Genes

A protein called leptin influences appetite, satiety, energy output and fertility, mainly via the hypothalamus, and it is now understood that leptin is influenced by a specific gene. The discovery of this 'obesity gene' led to great excitement as it seemed to be a let-out clause for fat people – 'I can't help it, it's in my genes'. However, it simply means that some people have a natural leaning towards fatness or, to put it another way, they just have to work harder at maintaining a healthy weight.

## Comfort eating

There must be very few people who have never sought solace in a glass of alcohol or a bar of chocolate, but when this becomes a regular habit, even an obsession, it becomes problematic. Bingeing and compulsive eating inevitably lead to weight gain, and obesity itself can become just another part of the problem that fuels the unhappiness.

## Quitting smoking

The last thing that should put you off giving up smoking is the worry about putting on weight. Yet weight gain is a common side-effect. Why? Nicotine dilates the blood vessels, allowing more blood to flow through, which includes the blood flow to the appetite centre in the hypothalamus. This keeps the appetite centre well supplied with glucose, suppressing the appetite. Cut off the effect of the nicotine and the appetite centre cries out for glucose, which is why so many people find they develop a craving for sugar. Smoking can also affect your metabolism; if your body metabolizes, or burns up, food less efficiently after you have given up smoking it will be more inclined to store the excess as fat.

## Chronic fatigue syndrome/ME

Two common symptoms of CFS are sugar cravings and very low energy levels, which both lead to weight problems. For more on CFS and its severe form, myalgic encephalomyelitis (ME), see page 272.

## Age

So often it comes as a nasty shock to find that, even though you eat no differently and are just as active, keeping to your ideal weight becomes more difficult as you get older – what you could get away with at 20 is no longer possible at 40 or 50. Many women also find they put on weight as they go through the menopause, and it is quite usual, as you reach old age, to gravitate either towards plumpness or skinniness.

## SMOKE AND LOSE WEIGHT?

There is a common but mistaken belief, especially among teenage girls, that smoking keeps you thin. It arises from the bizarre logic that if you put on weight when you stop smoking you must lose weight when you smoke. All it does, as explained above, is pave the way for hard-to-handle cravings when you later try to give up, as well as endanger your health.

## Alcohol

Many people still overlook alcohol as a source of excess weight, perhaps because it doesn't make us feel full and doesn't appear laden with the fats and sugars that we classically associate with fattening foods. But alcohol is not only high in energy (i.e. calories), it is easily absorbed, so that it quickly satisfies our body's energy requirements. This means that food we eat with it or later is largely seen as surplus to requirements in energy terms, and is stored away as fat.

## Prescription drugs

Certain drugs, such as steroids and some forms of HRT, are well known for causing weight gain, and even antidepressants and antibiotics taken over a long period can result in weight increase.

# WHAT'S THE PROBLEM?

## Family

Were your grandparents and parents (at least one from each generation) overweight or obese? **C**

Are your children overweight? (For an honest answer, ask other parents.) **C**

## Medical History

When you were born, was there anything that might have caused injury to the head or neck (forceps/ventouse delivery, ultra-rapid birth, slow birth over 24 hours)? **B**

Were you overweight as a child? (Compare yourself to the other children in old school photos rather than trusting your memory.) **C**

Have you ever had a fall that knocked you unconscious, broke your nose or injured your neck or skull? Or whiplash from a car accident? Or an accident as a child, such as a fall from a swing or tree, that jarred your neck? **B**

Did your weight problem begin at puberty? **B/C**

Do you suffer from endometriosis (see pages 104–6) or polycystic ovaries (see page 107)? **B**

Are you over 60? **D**

Are you prescribed thyroxine for a thyroid condition or have you been prescribed steroids for more than three months? **B**

Have you ever suffered from an eating disorder such as bulimia or obsessive-compulsive eating? **B**

Have you had a hysterectomy? **B**

Have you had a prolonged period of stress? (If this caused weight loss, answer A; if it caused weight gain, answer B/D) **A B/D**

## Habits

Do you always finish everything on your plate, perhaps out of politeness, even if you are not hungry? **C**

Do you often have a slice of cake, a biscuit or other small snack with tea or coffee? **D**

Are you in the habit of eating up the children's leftovers? **D**

Do you usually eat your main meal late in the evening? **D**

Do you find it particularly difficult to say no to cravings for particular foods, such as cream cakes or chocolate? **D**

Do you tend to eat more, or turn to specific comfort foods, when you are unhappy or bored? **D**

## Diet and Exercise

Do you succeed in losing weight if you go on a simple diet, such as low-fat or no meat? **A**

Do you lose weight if you give up specific high-calorie foods such as alcohol or butter and cream? **A**

Does even strict dieting make very little difference to your weight? **B**

**Do you lose weight on holiday if you do more swimming, walking, etc.?** A

**Do you lose weight if you take up a regular exercise regime?** A

**Do you put weight back on if you stop a diet or exercise regime?** A

**Have you always eaten sensibly but still gained weight?** B

**Does your excess fat accumulate especially on your thighs, hips and bottom, tummy, breasts and upper arms?** B

**Do you give yourself (or your family) food treats as a reward?** D

◆ **Did you answer Yes mostly to the A questions? That indicates that your main problem is one of eating too much and exercising too little.**
◆ **If you answered Yes to any B questions, then hormones will probably be playing a part in your weight problems. If you have a thyroid problem, or if your weight gain dates only since a hysterectomy or the menopause, it is probably the main cause.**
◆ **Any Cs? Then fat probably runs in the family, but you should consider carefully and honestly whether this is due to familial habits such as eating lots of big meals, rather than just blaming your genes.**
◆ **Answering Yes to D questions will have highlighted a psychological aspect to your eating habits, which can range from comfort eating in a small way to a real problem with your relationship to food.**

*Many women's weight problems stem from more than one cause.*

If you are overweight I suspect that you will have nodded in recognition at more than one of these brief descriptions. Perhaps reaching the menopause combined with a few too many sweet treats or boozy nights out? Or a sedentary life with too many opportunities to snack? Or a genetic predisposition to plumpness compounded by a long-standing family habit of large meals?

This short questionnaire (opposite) may help you to clarify things further.

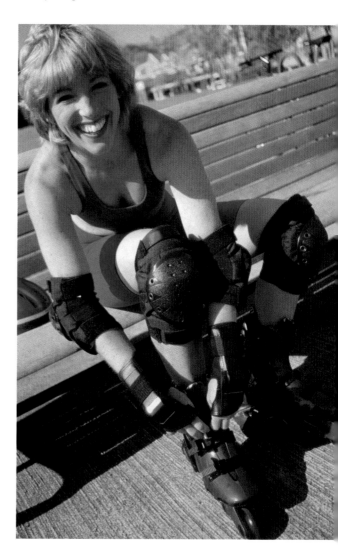

# Losing weight successfully
Before you start, weigh yourself and calculate what you should weigh (see box below). Your aim should be to lose about 1kg a week, and you may lose 500g or less a week.

Work out now roughly how long it is going to take to reach your target: it may seem a long stretch, but think of it as the path to a new, healthy life, not a sentence to be endured. Weight that falls off fast may boost morale but is also likely to come back all too quickly.

## WHAT SHOULD YOU WEIGH?

There is a formula that takes into account your height and weight to give an acceptable range into which you should fall. It is calculated as follows:

weight in kg ÷ height in metres$^2$
(measurements without clothes or shoes)

The answer is your Body Mass Index, or BMI. A BMI of 18.5–25 is normal, under 18 is usually considered underweight (see page 238), and 25 and higher is overweight. Over 30 is labelled obese (20 per cent or more above a healthy weight).

Examples:
51kg ÷ 1.7m$^2$ = 51 ÷ 2.89 = 17.6
57kg ÷1.6m$^2$ = 57 ÷ 2.56 = 22.2
76kg ÷ 1.64m$^2$ = 76 ÷ 2.7 = 28.1

To work out your acceptable weight range:
height$^2$ x 20 = lower weight in kg
height$^2$ x 25 = upper weight in kg

Also, measure your waist, hips and any areas, such as upper arms and thighs, where you would like to see a difference. Ratio of muscle to fat and weight distribution make a difference to your actual weight and shape, and when you reach a plateau in your weight loss (and most people do), you may find that you are continuing to shrink even though the scales seem stuck.

The most common cause of being overweight is eating too much and exercising too little, but as the questionnaire (page 224) will have highlighted, the reasons for this can be quite complex. Recognizing these underlying causes is an enormous help when it comes to losing weight. This applies especially to weight due to hormonal problems, which particularly afflict women. On pages 240–5 there is a special section on overcoming hormonally induced weight gain.

Whatever the reason for being overweight, solving the problem involves four elements:

■ nutrition

■ fasting

■ exercise

■ massage.

The constitution and balance of each of these will vary according to your type of overweight.

# Nutrition

For many years restrictive diets were based solely on calorific intake, and some still are. But you could limit yourself to, say, 1,000 calories a day by a 'diet' of two chocolate bars, a packet of crisps and a croissant, but it's not one to be advised!

## WHAT TO EAT

I do not recommend prescribed amounts of prescribed foods, so there is no 'diet plan' to follow here. What is important is rethinking the way you eat so that your dietary regime is just sufficient for your needs and as nutritious as possible, providing everything you need for optimum health and giving your body the tools to repair itself and resist ills.

Use the Nutrition section of the Lifestyle Programme as a guide to planning what you should include and what you should omit from your diet. In particular, you need to avoid foods that are going to increase your appetite or food cravings, or provide too much energy (too many calories) before you feel full. In particular, avoid:

◆ anything that increases stomach acid, and therefore appetite, including: acidic fruit, vinegary foods, over-spiced foods, scalding hot foods and drinks, deep-fried food, rough foods, such as nuts and seeds (if not chewed very well, these will increase your stomach acidity as it battles to break them down)
◆ too much yeast
◆ too much fat.

The simple food-combining guidelines described in the Lifestyle Programme – carbohydrates for breakfast to give a slow release of energy through the morning, protein and vegetables at lunchtime, and a lighter meal of carbohydrates and vegetables in the evening – are also helpful in food planning for weight loss.

## MEAL PLANNING

Sticking to the eating regime you have drawn up for yourself will be much easier with a little forethought.

◆ Sit down and plan the meals for the whole week. Resorting to takeaways or a last-minute dash to the shops is likely to conflict with your new regime.
◆ Draw up a shopping list – amounts as well as ingredients – from your meal plan and stick to it. Avoid impulse buys.
◆ It can be dispiriting to be faced with a long list of Don't Buys, so counter this with an equal list of Do Buys (see also Snack Attacks, see page 229).
◆ Take an objective look at how you shop. Think about taking frequent small shopping trips, which means fresh foods will be tastier and nutritionally better. Consider alternatives to supermarkets, thereby limiting the lure of being surrounded by foods on your Avoid list. Perhaps buying some food and non-consumables online will mean you have time to shop in local butchers, fishmongers and greengrocers instead – having to ask for each item individually is a good guard against impulse buying.
◆ Ban temptations such as cakes, sweets and crisps from the house, even if you are the only who needs to lose weight. Explain to the family why you are doing this and ask for their help.
◆ Institute regular mealtimes, so that you lessen the temptation to snack and your body becomes attuned to knowing when the next meal is arriving.

weight control

## HOW MUCH TO EAT

My grandfather always said: 'Stop eating when you feel you would be full if you had another mouthful,' which is good advice. There are two common factors in overeating:

■ eating too fast or not paying attention to what you are eating (see the box, Listen to Your Body)

■ habit. This often applies to families with a tendency to fatness – they have been brought up to think of the amount they eat as normal.

*If you think you fall into this second category:*

◆ assess your typical servings. An appropriate meat portion is about 75g or about the size of a pack of playing cards. How does this equate with yours? Count up how many starchy carbohydrate portions you consume in a day (see box below).

◆ check the amounts recommended in cookery books for meals you often eat; compare them with the amounts you use. If there is a discrepancy, this is a good indication that you should cut down. Psychologically, it may help to use smaller plates.

◆ avoid cooking more than you need. You then won't be tempted to eat up the leftovers. If you are intentionally cooking extra – more potatoes, say, for fishcakes the next day, or rice for a salad lunch tomorrow – then set this aside before you serve up and don't bring it to the table.

Eating too much can also be a psychological reaction to unhappiness or stress. Bingeing and compulsive eating disorder (see the chapter on Psychological Health) are extreme examples of this, but many people turn to food for comfort at bad times in their lives. Overfeeding your family, either at mealtimes or through constant sweet treats, can also be a way of compensating without realizing it – perhaps you find it difficult to express your love in other ways, or feel a need to 'prove' you don't neglect your children. These are difficult issues to deal with, but weight will continue to be a problem if the food link goes unrecognized.

On the other hand, it is not good to eat too little. If you consistently eat too little your body will read this as food being in short supply and go into 'famine mode' – which means it will endeavour to store fat even more efficiently.

## SERVING UP CARBOHYDRATES

The vast majority of the foods we eat contain carbohydrates in some form. There are two main types: sugars and starches. Fruits contain predominantly the sugar type (sugar itself is pure carbohydrate), cereal- or grain-based foods predominantly the starch type, and vegetables a varying mixture of the two.

Sugars, being simple in form, are quickly converted by the body into glucose and so bring swift relief from hunger, but the effects are short-lasting. The complex, starchy carbohydrates are digested more slowly and sustain us for longer. Just as we are advised to eat five portions of fruit and

vegetables every day, we should also include about six varied portions of starchy carbohydrates in our diet. Overestimating what constitutes a portion is a common way of eating too much.

1 portion =
◆ pasta/noodles: 3 rounded tbsp
◆ rice: 2 rounded tbsp
◆ bread: 1 thin slice
◆ potatoes: 1 medium
◆ breakfast cereal: 3 tbsp
◆ crackers or rice cakes: 3
◆ oatcakes: 2

## LISTEN TO YOUR BODY

Eat slowly and savour each mouthful, and your body will have time to send messages to your brain when it has had enough. If you bolt your food down these messages will arrive too late. When you are eating, concentrate on the food. If your mind is elsewhere – a TV programme, an engrossing book, on your work while lunching at your desk – it is easy to ignore your body's signals and eat too much. Also, you will not have received the benefit of enjoying your food, so soon you'll find yourself, not truly hungry, but yearning for a snack or another meal to provide the sensory satisfaction that comes from eating.

### WHEN TO EAT

Even choosing when you eat can help you lose weight. We are more likely to use up the energy we have taken in at breakfast and lunch than what we have for dinner, which is most often followed by a time of relaxing and sleeping. Yet for many people, dinner in the evening is the main meal of the day. And if you have skipped breakfast and had a hurried or snack lunch you are likely to feel very hungry by this time. To avoid hindering your bid to lose weight:

◆ Make lunch the main meal of the day if you can. This also coincides with the body's natural inner timetable, as it digests food most efficiently during the early afternoon. At night, while we sleep, is when it concentrates on renewing and repairing, so a heavy meal will take more of a toll on the body.

◆ If you have to have your main meal in the evening, try to eat early, say by 7 o'clock.

◆ Go for a walk after dinner, especially if this has been your main meal. This will stimulate your digestion and use up some of the energy that would otherwise be turned to fat.

◆ Try to stick to regular meal times and don't allow yourself to become ravenously hungry. An empty stomach tends towards acidity, sharpening your appetite.

## SNACK ATTACKS

Eating between meals on a regular basis is one of the most common reasons for weight gain. If you are cutting down on how much you eat, as well as revising what you eat, you are bound to get hunger pangs, at least until your stomach shrinks. Be realistic: you are not going to make the successful transition to your new eating regime if you are feeling constantly deprived or hungry and, of course, forbidden foods are all the more attractive. Prepare for this by taking evasive action:

| Instead of ... | choose |
| --- | --- |
| cakes or sweet biscuits | low-fat, low-sugar biscuits |
| sweets or chocolates | instant 'pop-in-the-mouth' fruit that needs no preparation: cherries, cape gooseberries (physalis), grapes, dates, blueberries |
| cheese | vegetables that can be eaten raw: mangetout, celery, carrots |
| creamy desserts | low-fat yoghurts |
| sweet or fizzy drinks | whole fruit juices (preferably non-citrus); flavoured mineral waters (they vary a lot in taste, so try out different ones – and experiment with adding your own flavouring) |

# Fasting

Incorporating a regular one-day fast and an occasional longer fast into your dietary regime is an effective way to help lose weight. A long fast is the most efficacious way to combat excess weight that is hormonal in origin, but this should only be done under medical supervision (see page 233).

## Do NOT fast if ...

**you are pregnant or suffer from any of the following: diabetes, heart disease, epilepsy, anaemia, very low blood pressure, kidney failure, osteoporosis, gout or stomach ulcers. Children should not fast unless they have been brought up in the tradition.**

### ONE-DAY FASTS

A pause in your food intake once a week is an excellent aid in a weight-loss plan. As well as having the obvious advantage of reducing the overall amount you eat each week, it refreshes your palate and helps you appreciate your food more, rather than taking it for granted. It is also of general benefit to your body and mind.

Choose a specific day each week to fast, taking into account the rhythm of your life. Monday may be a good day, to compensate for any excesses over the weekend, or a day when work is not too demanding, or a Saturday or Sunday if these are days when you have more time. Pick a day when you can relax and pamper yourself a little: make it a rewarding day, not a punishment.

Although you are giving your body a rest from food, don't restrict your fluid intake. Make sure you drink plenty of water (at least 1½ litres), which can be either plain or flavoured (see Vital Fluids box on page 232).

Not everyone can go 24 hours without any food at all. If you have a very active or stressful life, or if you find that your moods become difficult to control, or you feel light-headed or weak, then opt for a semi-fast rather than giving up the idea. Allow yourself one of the following and see which suits you best:

◆ a portion of fresh fruit first thing in the morning and two or three more portions during the day as you feel you need it. Avoid citrus fruit and too much other acidic fruit such as kiwi, passion fruit or pineapple. Melon, grapes, cherries, apples, pears, plums, peaches and apricots are all good choices. Avoid bananas as they have a high glycaemic index. Freshly juiced vegetables: try carrot, celery, mint, beetroot or cucumber, either on their own or in combinations.

◆ home-made vegetable soup (see recipe below): a bowl at lunchtime and another early evening.

Don't prepare yourself by eating double the day before!

## VEGETABLE SOUP

**Bring 1½ litres of water to the boil in a large saucepan. Add a selection of chopped vegetables: cabbage, broccoli and other brassicas, carrots, peas, onions, leeks and courgettes are all good, but don't include potatoes. Add those that take longest to cook first, and simmer gently until all the vegetables are soft. Blend the mixture to make a thick but easily digested soup.**

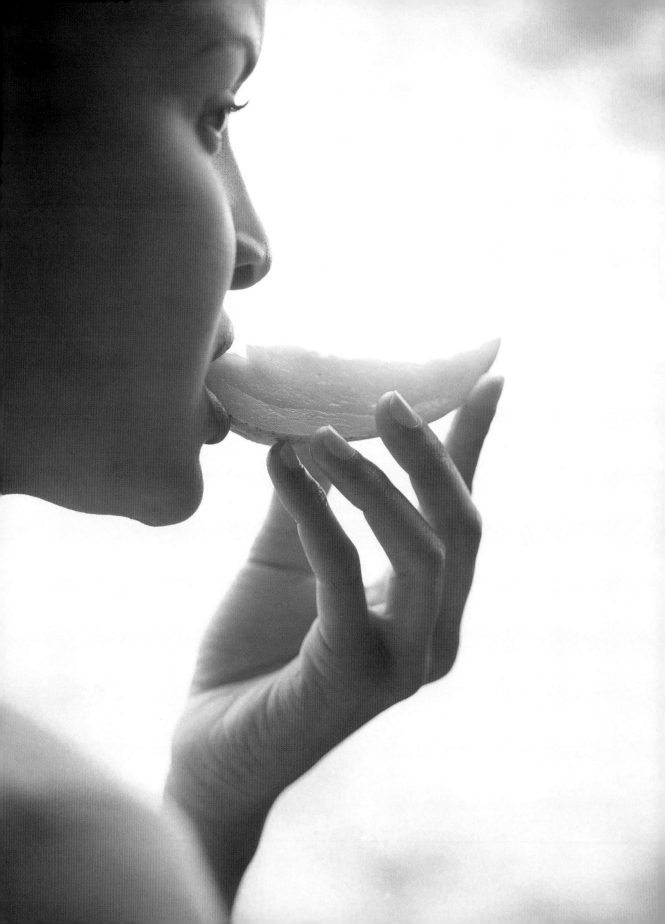

## THREE-DAY FASTS

Perhaps twice a year, a three-day fast can give your body a real boost. It can put you back on the straight and narrow if you have lapsed over a celebratory period, such as Christmas or a family wedding, and it provides your body with an extended chance to adjust to eating less.

A three-day fast follows much the same pattern as a one-day fast, but because of its longer duration you will need to plan it a little more carefully.

◆ Choose a period when you can devote at least Days 2 and 3 to relaxation (you can work on Day 1 if you need to, although it is preferable not to).

◆ Plan a light meal for the evening before your fast and for the day after. Buy the ingredients for these, for vegetable soup on your last evening (see Vegetable Soup box) and for alternatives to plain water (see Vital Fluids box).

◆ Make arrangements so that you do not need to go shopping or cook for others during your fast.

◆ Ensure you have to hand everything you need to encourage relaxation and pass the time quietly but without getting bored: your favourite soft music, a good book, massage oils, aromatic candles …

◆ Unless you live on your own, enlist flatmates, partner or family to help make this a relaxing time for you.

◆ The evening before, make up fasting tea, and lime and honey water (see box), both of which will provide some sustenance as well as a welcome alternative to plain water.

## VITAL FLUIDS

Throughout a fast you should ensure that you have sufficient fluids, at least 1½ litres a day. Ring the changes from plain water with a calming herbal tea such as chamomile, fasting tea, and lime and honey water. Prepare these last two beforehand so that they are readily to hand.

**Fasting tea**
In a saucepan put 1½ litres of water, 6 cloves, 2 cinnamon sticks and 1 tablespoon of aniseed. If you like you may also add 2 tablespoons of dried cranberries. Boil together for five minutes and leave to infuse before straining.

**Lime and honey water**
Warm 2 tablespoons of honey so that it flows easily and stir it into 2 litres of water. Add the freshly squeezed juice of half a lime (not more, or the water will be over-acidic).

### The evening before
Begin to wind down your food intake with a light meal: vegetable soup and some salad, or steamed vegetables with rice or pasta.

### Day 1
Water and fasting tea. You may work on this day.

### Day 2
Water and fasting tea. No work. Sleep as much as you can and pass the day in the relaxed way you have planned. A massage and a couple of steam baths or hot soaks are essentials, as you will feel tired.

### Day 3
As Day 2, but break your fast in the evening with some vegetable soup.

### Day 4

Reintroduce yourself gently to food again; don't shock your body. Have some fruit and perhaps porridge for breakfast, and a light lunch and dinner similar to your meal the evening before your fast. Eat slowly and enjoy the enhanced flavour that food seems to have – after your period of abstinence your sense of taste and smell will be sharper and more finely tuned.

As you become used to fasting you can increase the fasting time in stages, and under the supervision of a qualified naturopath, up to a maximum of seven days. No liquid-only fast should extend beyond this without close medical supervision and on approved premises.

## LONGER FASTS

Correctly monitored, a long fast can have amazing results in overcoming weight gain that is hormonal in origin. In depriving your body of food, it naturally turns to its own reserves, i.e. the stores of fat it has accumulated for just this sort of (as your body sees it) crisis. If the root cause of your overweight is hormonal, much of the excess fat will be white fat, or cellulite (see box, page 240). The body does not look upon these cellulite deposits as its primary source of energy, so they will not diminish while there is still plenty of yellow fat to rely on. A long fast, of three weeks or so, forces the body to draw on these cellulite reserves for sustenance.

### How a long fast works

Deprived of food, the body reacts in a series of stages. For the first three days or so, there are the expected hunger pangs, fatigue and dreams of food. Then, miraculously, these sensations disappear, to be followed by a week of buoyant well-being – it has been observed that conditions such as eczema and swollen joints improve noticeably during this period. Then, between the seventh and ninth day of fasting the healing crisis occurs. Everything gets much worse, and patients are confined to bed to receive lots of fluids and light massage, and possibly enemas or colonic irrigation; a glucose drip may be necessary.

A couple of days later the patients emerge from the crisis calm, clear-eyed and feeling in excellent health. The fast continues for a further week, which they experience in a happy and creative frame of mind. There is elation at the weight lost and great motivation to continue with the dietary regime, strengthened by the sense of having successfully endured a difficult journey. After fasting, the return to food is managed slowly, beginning with soft bland foods that are easy to digest. A welcome side-effect is the sharply accentuated sense of taste.

The care of a qualified physician experienced in fasting therapy is paramount throughout this process, to assess mental attitude and to monitor and understand the bodily changes that occur – blood tests during the healing crisis show bizarre readings, liver enzymes rise and kidney function alters. There are fasting specialists in Germany, Russia, India and the United States, and I am planning my own specialized fasting therapy at our proposed sanitorium in London.

# Exercise

Weight control is a matter of balance. If you consume more than your body requires, it will convert the excess into fat deposits. Athletes in training, polar explorers and anyone doing a lot of physical work will consume a lot of high-energy food and yet not put on weight because their bodies are using up all they eat and more. Similarly, if the height of daily activity is picking up the telephone or loading the dishwasher, then even a starvation diet will mean more energy is being taken in than expended.

Being overweight can make it more difficult to exercise sufficiently to reduce those fat stores – and so you find yourself in a vicious circle that must be broken.

## GETTING STARTED

If you are very overweight, or have not done any exercise for a very long time, have yourself assessed at a well-woman clinic, by your GP or a qualified fitness trainer with experience of developing programmes for people who are out of condition. Launching into an inappropriate self-imposed regime could do more harm than good and could put your heart and lungs as well as muscles and joints under dangerous strain.

The early days may be very modest – a walk around the local park each morning or perhaps just a short session of exercises while sitting down – but regularity is important, and so is building up the amount you do. Work to a structured plan so that your level of exercise is increasing safely but steadily in line with your stamina and muscular tone.

## WHICH EXERCISE?

'Exercise' may conjure up for you an image of lithe ladies in leg-warmers or sweaty joggers on the streets at dawn, or other scenarios you would cringe from joining. Thankfully, there are plenty of alternatives. Choose something that suits you, so that you are not forever finding excuses to avoid it. Here are just a few ideas:

- **Yoga** I particularly favour yoga, which is especially suitable if you are overweight. You can do it in the privacy of your own home if you wish, it does not put unnecessary strain on your body and from simple breathing and stretching techniques develops into a strenuous and demanding workout. For more on yoga, see pages 76–81.

# BODY FAT: THE GOOD AND THE BAD

Our bodies cannot do without fat. It provides us with the greatest part of our energy but also, among other things, cushions our vital organs against shock, protects the breast glands that produce milk and helps our eyes move easily.

Rather as a camel is able to store fat in its hump, we have evolved to store energy in the form of fat. We derive our energy from what we eat, and when we eat more than our body needs for the moment, it stores rather than wastes this potential energy. When our ancestors were never sure where the next meal might be coming from, this was a life-saving trick that we have never lost and it is still needed today. Should we need an unexpected burst of energy – to run from danger, or play a spontaneous game of catch with the children, for instance – it means we don't have to sit down and eat something first.

However, one can have too much of a good thing. If we habitually consume more than we 'burn off', our deposits of fat will get greater and greater.

## EVERYDAY ENERGY

Remember that, as far as your body is concerned, anything that calls on its energy reserves will help reduce fat deposits, not just something labelled 'exercise'. So look also at your ordinary daily activity: take the stairs instead of the lift at work; walk a friend's dog or baby; attack household chores like vacuuming, cleaning the windows or mowing the lawn with extra vigour. And singing as you do it consumes even more energy!

■ **Swimming** Being buoyed up in the water relieves pressure on your joints and gives you a great sense of freedom from your own weight. Find out about sessions specifically for your age or weight group so you are not put off by hordes of children or serious swimmers in training. As well as swimming, many pools are used for aquaerobics and similar water-based exercises.

■ **Dancing** More and more, dance is being recognized as beneficial exercise as well as being enjoyable. And not just the overtly energetic forms: ballroom dancing, for example, is a wonderful muscle toner and improves stamina and breathing.

■ **Walking** Everyone should try to do more walking.

■ **Tai chi** This gentle yet invigorating exercise is actually a form of martial art, but, like yoga, its graduated development and emphasis on co-ordinated, unstrained movements make it a good choice even for the obese.

There are many classes run especially for the overweight (you'll probably find you are far from the largest person

there), and as well as providing suitably pitched exercise they often act as an informal support group – sharing experiences and encouragement is good for morale and will help you through difficult patches.

If this is not an option or you are too embarrassed by your size, videos and DVDs abound on almost every subject – set aside time each day to follow a regime in front of the TV, just like an educational course.

## Massage

In the Lifestyle Programme, I explain the value of massage. If you are trying to lose weight, it can help by:

◆ relieving stress (reducing the chances of stress-induced cravings or over-eating)
◆ improving mood, helping you feel positive and reinforcing your determination to lose weight
◆ improving blood flow to the hypothalamus, which regulates the appetite centre and hormonal balance.

Incorporate a weekly neck massage into your weight-loss plan. It is possible to do this yourself, but easier and more effective to enlist the help of a partner or friend.

## Other aids

◆ Gokhru tea is helpful in reducing fluid retention.
◆ Chawanprash is a traditional mixture of plant extracts that is rich in minerals, vitamins and other nutrients, and can be a useful form of supplement while you are on a restricted diet.
◆ A good multivitamin/mineral formulation will help boost your energy levels.

## REACHING A PLATEAU

Typically weight loss follows a stop-start pattern:

◆ an encouraging initial loss
◆ a slower loss of about 1kg or less a week
◆ a plateau when, whatever you do, your weight refuses to drop any further.

Keep with your initial plan for at least 12 weeks. When after that you get stuck at the same spot for two weeks, keep to the same dietary regime but increase your level of exercise. You are now able to sustain a greater level of activity, and increasing your body's metabolic rate by more intense exercise will mean it draws on its fat reserves at a greater rate.

When you reach a second plateau you should have reached the maximum potential for this plan. You should now continue with a sensible life-long eating, exercise and massage pattern as outlined in the Lifestyle Programme.

# Keeping the weight at bay Once you have lost your excess weight, the last thing you will want to do is put it back on again.

Because you have lost it at a slow rate and retrained your body and eating habits at the same time, you are unlikely to regain it, but keep a check on your weight and measurements, so that any weight increase doesn't creep up on you unawares.

careful not to undo all the good work. Modify your strict diet slowly, introducing small amounts of fat or carbohydrate until you are eating in the style outlined in the Lifestyle Programme (page 63). Eating moderately and balancing diet with exercise and massage will be important for the rest of your life.

## Nutrition

You may find, like many of my patients, that following the guidelines at the beginning of this chapter has transformed your way of eating forever. Or you may feel irked by certain deprivations. These can probably safely be reintroduced into your diet in moderation – try one thing at a time, as you may find your body responds differently to some things after a long abstinence.

Most people find that simply listening to their body's eating requirements as they have learnt to do, combined with daily exercise and weekly massage, is sufficient to keep their weight at a sensible and healthy level. Maintaining the practice of a one-day fast once a week is beneficial and you can compensate for any over-indulgence with a stricter regime or semi-fast for a few days.

If you have been through the tough regime for hormonal overweight, you will need to be particularly

## Exercise and massage

As you lose weight and your level of fitness improves, ever more exercise options will become available to you. When, perhaps for much of your life, you have thought of yourself as 'a fat person' it can be difficult to shake off the image in your mind even when you have lost a lot of weight.

Open your mind to new possibilities: different sports such as fencing; joining a tennis club; perhaps even training to teach others or help coach children.

Keeping a weekly massage is a worthwhile part of your routine; do not think of it as self-indulgence. All the help it has been along the way – calming and relaxing you, improving the performance of your hypothalamus – will continue to be of assistance and reduce still further your chances of going back to your old ways and old weight.

# If you are underweight Far fewer people suffer from being underweight than overweight, but if you do it is no less of a worry.

Other women, who struggle to keep their weight down, probably have little sympathy and may even be envious, but being underweight brings its own problems.

Serious loss of weight may be symptomatic of illness or disease, so it is always important that you get a full check-up at the surgery or hospital. Assuming that there is no underlying illness, check out what and how much you are eating. Eating too little over a sustained period can have the effect of:

◆ nutritional deficiencies from an incomplete diet
◆ weakening the immune system, encouraging frequent colds and coughs
◆ low energy and stamina, and general aches and pains
◆ anaemia or low blood pressure, causing fatigue, dizziness, nausea, headaches, fainting bouts, breathlessness, etc.
◆ fertility problems
◆ increased risk of osteoporosis.

If you have a naturally fast metabolism (not caused by an overactive thyroid) or your appetite is gone, you could try the following to maximize your nutrition and increase your energy:

◆ Mashed banana and cream with a little honey, after breakfast.
◆ About 1 tablespoon of ghee stirred into a dish of rice or lentils. This form of clarified butter provides a high level of nourishment as it is 'potentized' by thorough churning that breaks down its component parts, making it easily digested and absorbed.

◆ Lean red meat with a lot of salad (lettuce, onions, radishes, tomatoes) to aid its digestion.
◆ Sufficient fats in healthy forms: avocados, nuts and seeds, nut butters, olive oil and oil-rich fish.
◆ Home-made marrowbone stock. Simmer marrowbones from organic lamb or beef shanks for two hours with garlic, ginger, nutmeg, cinnamon sticks, bay leaves and whole peppercorns. (You can make up a quantity of this, strain it and keep it in individual portions in the freezer.) Drink a mug of stock about an hour before your main meal.
◆ Potatoes, pasta and porridge: all good sources of carbohydrates that aid weight gain.
◆ Kefir: this Russian/Eastern European preparation similar to yoghurt is fermented and processed in a particular way; the churning process it undergoes breaks the bond between the amino acids, making them easily absorbed and synthesized into protein in the body.
◆ Ashwagandha (Indian ginseng): this is a powerful adaptogen (i.e. it helps the body adapt to stress) and helps to build up energy and muscle bulk.

# Appetite stimulants

## A FEW SUGGESTIONS

◆ 1 teaspoon of brandy in warm water or a small
   sherry
◆ 1 teaspoon of jal jeera, a traditional Indian appetite
   enhancer of cumin, tamarind and black salt, in a
   glass of water
◆ drakshasava – an ayurvedic balsam made from
   grapes and herbs into a weak alcoholic drink that
   stimulates appetite and aids digestion.

Drink one of these half an hour before a meal.

Additionally, help your body to relax with a twice-
weekly massage with a calming aromatherapy oil (see
page 69) and the 'salutation to the sun' yoga routine
(see pages 78–9).

**See also Anorexia in the chapter on Psychological
Health, pages 258–61.**

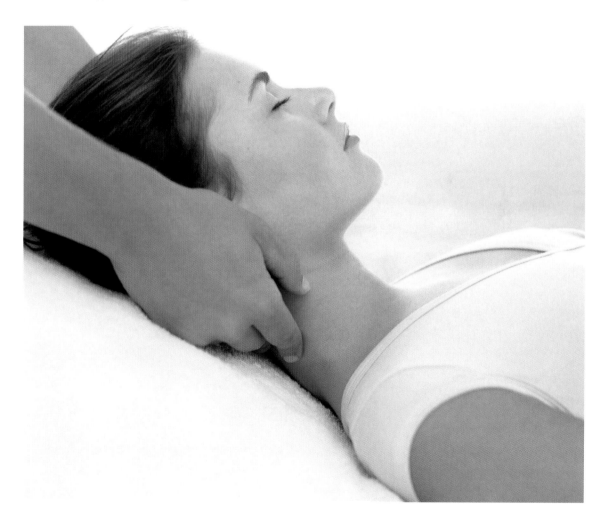

# Conquering hormonal weight gain For a significant minority of women, obesity is caused predominantly by a hormonal imbalance.

This leads to a build-up of white fat, or cellulite (see box). Weight gain linked to the menopause is also often of this hormonally induced variety.

Whereas an ordinary weight-loss regime works by reducing your reserves of body fat, the aim in correcting hormonal weight gain is to trigger a biochemical change that breaks down cellulite fat and improves hormonal balance.

The most effective way to do this is a long fast, of around three weeks, which forces your body to turn to its reserves of white fat for the nourishment it needs to survive (see page 233). There are currently very few places where you can go and safely undertake this fasting therapy, which needs to be done in a clinic under expert supervision, so this is the plan I suggest to patients who come to me with weight problems that are predominantly hormonal. It is their lasting success that has proved that, with determination and patience, this is a programme that works.

**STAGE 1**

■ A three-day fast (see pages 232–3).

**STAGE 2**

■ Follow either the minimal-fat diet (see page 242) or the high-protein, low-fat, low-starch diet (see pages 244–5) for at least six months, preferably longer. The first couple of weeks are the hardest, after which you begin to enjoy a new way of eating.

■ A one-day fast once a week.

■ Weekly neck massage (see page 66) to help improve blood flow to the hypothalamus, which controls hormonal output and also fluid retention, which may be adding to your weight. Direct massage of the affected areas is also beneficial).

## YELLOW FAT AND WHITE FAT

**Yellow fat** is 'ordinary' fat, the stores our body has created from what we have eaten but not used up. It can be deposited not only on hips and buttocks, stomachs, limbs and cheeks, but around the heart and intestines and other organs.

**White fat** is commonly called cellulite and most typically appears on the thighs and buttocks as an unattractive dimpling effect. It is created when a hormonal imbalance in a woman's body has led to

an excess of male hormones. As a protective reaction, the body converts these into oesterone, a female hormone resembling oestrogen. This 'spare but safe' hormone is then stored in white fat, which can appear not only on the thighs and buttocks, but also the breasts, upper arms and waist. Since cellulite is a repository of excess hormones rather than excess energy, it responds poorly to the sort of diet and exercise regime that reduces yellow fat.

# PREPARATION

**Prepare yourself mentally for a tough regime for at least six months, and for a lifelong change to the way you eat. This takes tremendous will-power, so be ready to use whatever works best for you in achieving mind over matter, be it prayer, meditation or yoga relaxation techniques.**

**There will be times when your resolve will weaken, but if you give in the process has to begin again from the beginning – because this involves altering your body's biochemistry you cannot simply compensate for a day's lapse by trying extra hard the next day.**

■ An exercise regime. This may need to be very gentle at first if you are very overweight and out of condition, so take professional advice. Not all your excess weight will be white fat, so your yellow fat will begin to reduce with exercise.

### STAGE 3

■ Continue to follow the plan outlined in the Lifestyle Programme of diet, massage and exercise. As you have a tendency towards hormonally induced fat, you will need to stick to a sensible regime for the rest of your life.

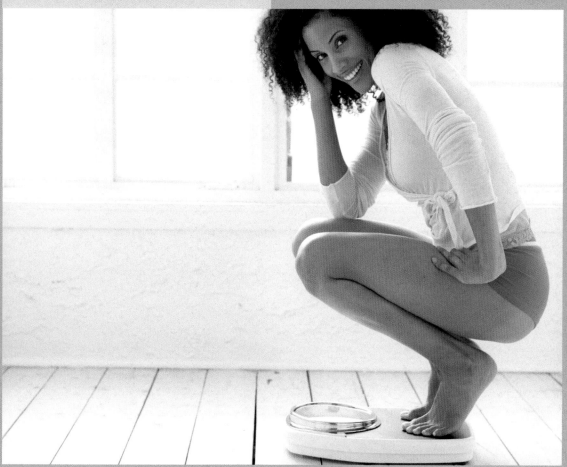

# The minimal-fat diet

For this, you need to cut out all fats and the majority of oils, so that your body has to turn to its reserves, which includes cellulite, not only to fuel your every activity but to manufacture the essential fatty acids and cholesterol to keep your basic systems functioning.

Protein and carbohydrate levels can remain normal – but check that your usual portions are normal and not oversized (see How much to eat, page 228).

**NB: Restricting your proteins and carbohydrates as well can speed up weight loss, but this is a diet that puts the body under great strain anyway, so do not cut back on these other two food groups as well for longer than three months. Impose too great a burden on yourself and you are more likely to give up.**

*Foods to avoid:*
- all meat except the lowest-fat types (see below)
- all dairy products except small amounts of low-fat yoghurts and some low-fat milk for cereal and tea
- fats and oils in cooking or for dressings or sauces, except very small amounts of vegetable or olive oils.

*Permitted in moderation:*
- nuts
- eggs
- oily fish (comparatively high in fat, but of a type necessary for health), without the skin

This may look at first quite manageable, but as you plan your meals you will realize just how much we rely on fats in one form or another for cooking and flavouring. You will miss the unctuousness and satisfying sense of fullness fat gives. Fat also adds taste, so explore different ways of making meals as flavourful as possible (see Maximizing Flavour, opposite).

## LOW-FAT MEATS

### Choose:
- **organic chicken and turkey (without the skin)** recent studies show fat levels in average chickens are much higher than they used to be
- **lean game birds (i.e. partridge, pheasant breast; but not duck or goose)**
- **venison**
- **lamb's kidney**
- **veal fillet**
- **extra-lean ham**
- **ostrich**
- **pork fillet**
- **rabbit**
- **lean rump steak**

In time, a bland diet will re-educate your tastebuds, which have probably been dulled by decades of multiple taste sensations in the same meal, to appreciate subtle nuances of flavour, but be as inventive as you can within the diet's restrictions to help you stay the course.

Be wary of reduced-fat preparations: the label can just mean 'lower than usual', or indicate the use of fat substitutes that may affect our bodies in ways of which we are unaware. Try to avoid where possible.

## MEAL IDEAS

### Breakfast
- cottage cheese with crushed walnuts or cashew nuts
- oatmeal porridge cooked with half water, half soya or low-fat milk
- fresh fruit
- boiled or poached egg, from time to time

Although bread is permitted, it is perhaps not a good choice if you can't do without accompaniments like butter and spreads (you could try low-fat cottage cheese).

## Lunch/dinner

- plenty of vegetables and a complex carbohydrate (such as rice, potatoes or pasta) with a portion of low-fat meat or fish or a vegetarian equivalent such as tofu

For protein, in addition to the suggestions above, expand your repertoire with:

- white fish
- shellfish (except crab)
- high-protein pulses, such as black-eye beans, lentils and kidney beans

## COPING WITHOUT FAT

To replace the rich smoothness missing from a minimal-fat diet:

- thick soups based on lentils or dried beans (these are both filling and creamy smooth).
- nuts: chew them well, so as not to encourage your stomach to increase its acidity, and again, eat them only in moderation. Their oils line the stomach to give a satisfactory sensation of fullness.

## MAXIMIZING FLAVOUR

Meals without fat or oil tend to be very bland, but avoid the temptation of adding more salt or sugar in an effort to lift the taste. Most of your cooking will be steaming, baking and boiling, so experiment with the myriad different herbs and spices available (only avoiding very hot chillies, as these are appetite enhancers), using them in different ways.

Marinate meat, fish and vegetarian substitutes such as tofu and soya cubes before cooking – here are just a few ideas for marinades:

- fresh tomatoes, onions, garlic, ginger and mustard, blended or ground to a pulp
- crushed garlic and dill (good with fish)
- a mix of curry spices and flavourings such as ginger, garlic, cinnamon, cardamom, cloves and a little turmeric
- finely chopped fresh coriander leaves, crushed garlic and a little grated lemon zest.

Other flavour-enhancing ideas:

- Make a stuffing, with a base of breadcrumbs bound together with a little beaten egg white. Add pepper, a little salt and whatever flavouring you like; you could include a few finely crushed nuts too. Use it to fill slits cut in poultry, or the cavity of a whole fish, or as a filling for parcels or rolls of thin fillets
- Bake en papillote: before cooking in the oven, seal fish or meat in a foil or greaseproof paper parcel with sprigs of fresh herbs (orange or lemon thyme is very good with fish; marjoram with chicken), a little sea salt and black pepper. Cooking this way infuses the flesh with the flavourings and keeps it succulent as no juices escape. A variation on this is to use leaves as a wrap: try vine, cabbage or large sorrel leaves
- Grill or barbecue meat and fish over sprigs of herbs such as rosemary, fennel, thyme, or stalks of lemon grass
- Add finely chopped spring onions and/or herbs to mashed potato or other puréed root vegetables
- A little squeeze of fresh lemon or lime juice is a good flavour lifter.

# The high-protein, low-starch diet

I must stress straight away that this is not the same as the high-protein, high-fat, low-carbohydrate diet popular in recent years. In the regime I am detailing here, starchy carbohydrates and fats are kept low – the body is forced to rely on its fat reserves – so this is one that can safely be followed over a long period and is an effective way of losing weight that stems from a hormonal imbalance if followed for at least six months, preferably a year.

In the main your energy and nutrition will be coming from 250–400g of foods such as fish, meat, eggs, which are high in protein, with plenty of leafy vegetables and fruit.

## ROUGHAGE

Cutting grains, pulses, etc., from your diet also reduces the fibre or roughage you are eating, but it is important not to become constipated. Many fruits provide good levels of roughage, but ensure you also get as much 'neutral' roughage as you can (i.e. from sources that are not high in sugars) by eating plenty of leafy green vegetables.

Other useful counters to constipation are:

- **psyllium husks:** 1–2 teaspoons stirred into water and swallowed quickly before they set, and followed by more water
- **papaya:** the natural enzyme papain aids digestion of protein and has a mild laxative effect
- **Chawanprash:** this traditional Indian tonic (see page 235) aids elimination as well as being full of nutrients.

If necessary, take a mild senna laxative occasionally, to ease the bowels.

## FOODS TO AVOID

The principal foods to cut from your diet are the starchy carbohydrates:

- bread
- pasta and noodles
- rice and other grains, including sweetcorn
- beans, peas and lentils
- potatoes and other starchy root vegetables
- squashes (pumpkins and their relations)
- frozen peas
- breakfast cereals

Nuts and seeds vary a lot in their fat and starchy carbohydrate content. Avoid:

- chestnuts
- cashews
- peanuts

You should also reduce your fat intake, although not as drastically as in the minimal-fat diet (see page 242–3). In particular, avoid:

- butter
- cheese
- cream
- fatty meats

## MEAL IDEAS

### Breakfast
- boiled or poached egg
- fresh fruit
- fruit smoothie made with low-fat milk
- yoghurt
- tea

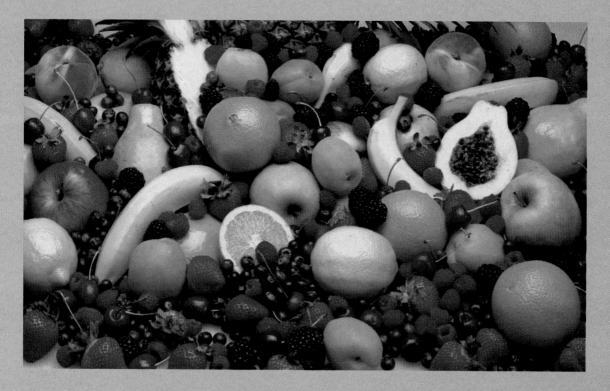

### Lunch/dinner

◆ grilled lean meat with stir-fried vegetables

◆ casseroled poultry or game (not duck or goose) with a selection of vegetables added towards the end of the cooking time or steamed and served separately

◆ fish, grilled or baked

◆ Japanese-style soup with plenty of vegetables and strips of meat and/or fish and/or tofu poached in a flavourful clear broth

◆ fresh fruit for dessert

### Tips when devising meals ...

◆ As a guide, the daily protein you should be eating equates to about two meaty chicken thighs or two thick steaks of fish.

◆ Marinating meat, fish or tofu adds flavour and interest. There are some ideas in the minimal-fat diet (page 242–3), and you can expand the repertoire with yoghurt or olive oil.

◆ Fruit such as bananas and mangoes might contribute to weight gain on a normal regime, but are not a problem when you have cut out so much else, so enjoy them and benefit from their nutritional content.

◆ Salad vegetables eaten raw, such as lettuce, rocket, celery, watercress and spring onions help with protein digestion.

◆ Ridding rice of much of its starch means it is possible to make it part of a meal from time to time. Wash the rice thoroughly (you will see the water is at first cloudy with released starch), then boil it in plenty of water (don't steam it), then transfer to a sieve and rinse again thoroughly with fresh boiling water.

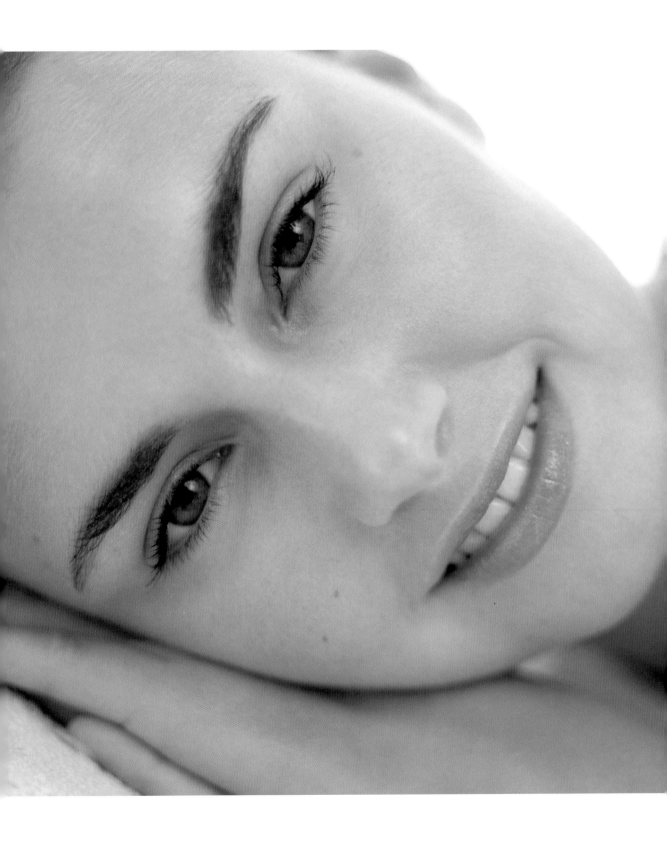

# chapter eight

# psychological health

In developing countries the major threats to health come from disease, malnutrition and public hygiene. Conversely, in highly developed countries illness is compounded, not by lack of medical help but by the stress of everyday living. The state of our mind affects our body, somtimes in a direct, traumatic way, such as deep shock causing hair to turn white or fall out, but usually in much more insidious and subtle ways. Workaholics may find themselves vulnerable to any bug that's floating around; unhappiness or low self-esteem can lead to eating disorders; fretting about not getting pregnant can make conception more difficult.

# Stresses and strains Being in a constant state of nervous worry or tension is obviously detrimental to your health, but stress is on the increase.

## Actions and reactions

Stress is a natural reaction of the body. When faced with a threat or a dilemma, the body automatically gears up to respond in a way that prepares it to face the problem or run away: fight or flight. That is why an athlete in a race and an actor waiting to perform on stage can experience much the same symptoms: a faster-beating heart, sweating, tense muscles and increased breathing and metabolic rate. When the moment is over, the symptoms calm down and everything returns to normal.

But when a stress-inducing situation doesn't resolve itself so simply and becomes a feature or regular occurrence of our everyday life, stress becomes a conditioned reflex. We have all the symptoms of 'fight or flight' without the calming aftermath. The body remains in a state of alertness most of the time, wasting energy and heightening our level of tension. Such pathological stress is harmful, because the body is allowed no time to recuperate. It's like flying a plane without carrying out maintenance in between flights: the performance slows down and the danger of breakdown increases.

Factors as varied as long-haul flights or processing alcohol put greater strain on a woman's body than on a man's, and if you do not get your balance of life right it will put your mind and your body under stress that can be damaging.

What sort of things should you be aware are likely to cause this harmful type of stress?

## A JUGGLING ACT

The pressures on a woman are multiple throughout her life, from doing well at school to finding a boyfriend; 'proving herself' in a challenging career, or feeling she has to justify being 'just a housewife'; keeping on top of home and work life while satisfying demands from family and friends; coming to terms with getting older and fighting off or disguising the signs of ageing. Many women feel they are involved in a constant juggling act.

Despite apparent equality, women often carry greater responsibilities in a family – more often than not it is she rather than her partner who has to take time off work when the children are ill, or on whom the practicalities of looking after elderly parents fall. At work, concession is seldom made for this double life. While these demands make you adept at dealing with any type of difficulty thrown your way, it may mean you fail to recognize problems brewing inside yourself.

## EMOTIONAL STRAIN

Each emotion has its own special centre in the brain, most being located in the limbic system. There is still much to learn about how these centres correlate, but we can see the effects in bodily changes. Embarrassment can make us blush; fear or bad news can make us vomit, lose control of our bowels or faint. Your heart may throb with passion or melt with sympathy, or your hair may stand on end in fright: these are clichéd expressions but ones that show we recognize that emotions cause our body as well as our mind to react.

These chemical responses have their own 'half-life' – it takes a while for the muscle tension of anger or the trembling of fear to subside. Reaction times vary from person to person, but if your body is subjected to successive waves of emotional highs it doesn't have time to come back down in between. A state of tension comes to feel like the norm. Such tension does not have to be a major threat, such as your life in danger or having lost your home and loved ones, but exists in the persistent low-level worry of feeling you're out of your depth at work or unhappy in a relationship.

## DILEMMAS AND DECISIONS

If a hungry donkey is put between two stacks of hay, it finds it difficult to decide which one to eat first. Having to make choices can make us similarly stall and be unable to move forward. Stress builds up.

A certain amount of stress helps our bodies and brains perform better and enables us to achieve things we couldn't before. Too much stress, though, especially if it is caused by something being thrust upon us unexpectedly or something totally beyond our

## EMOTIONAL TELEPATHY

Emotions can also be affecting at one remove. Just like animals, we pick up on positive and negative emotions, even though this may be subconscious. Emotions don't have to be communicated verbally: body language, eye contact, gestures or even lack of communication all convey mood and emotion. Living or working in close proximity to negative emotion is bound to create a lot of tension, the worse for feeling it is beyond your control because nothing has been said – it may not even be directed at you.

experience, can have an adverse effect. We react with anxiety, depression, irritability, aggression, or may even have a nervous breakdown.

## CHANGE

When change is unwanted and not within your control, it can cause great worry and tension. Redundancy from work, a forced move, or divorce are all obvious examples.

It is common for people to get set in their ways as they get older, and so become more resistant to change and vulnerable to its stresses. If you have spent your whole adult life building a busy career, or caring for a demanding family, or both, retirement or becoming an 'empty nester' as your family leaves home can come as a shock.

To begin with, the lack of routine and pressures may seem like a marvellous luxury. But if you have not allowed yourself interests of your own you may find yourself at a loss. Some women who have devoted themselves unstintingly to their family are hit hard by a sense of no longer being indispensable. Turning from mother to grandmother can be a fulfilling new role, but with today's widely scattered families this is not always an option. Others, whose life has been solely work-orientated, feel isolated if they know few of their neighbours or have little in common with them. Lethargy, depression, alcoholism, eating disorders and hypochondria are all possible outcomes.

# Stress management Working more hours than ever before, and not making the best use of our leisure time has meant stress levels are at an all-time high.

## Conserving energy

Stress is very energy-draining. And when you lack energy your body copes less well: you are less able to fend off minor illnesses, take longer to recuperate, you think less clearly, and problems, especially emotional ones, assume disproportionate dimensions.

Think about how you spend a typical week. Can things be made easier?

■ Are there tasks you do out of habit rather than necessity?

■ Do you have to do them, or could they fall to someone else?

■ Many women dismiss the idea of employing a cleaner, and not always for reasons of cost; often it can be because they feel guilty at the thought of paying someone else to do 'their' work, something they could do just as easily themselves. If you can afford some help with housework, you should look at it as buying yourself time – don't use this time to catch up on more work, or do the shopping. Instead go swimming, walking, take a painting class or anything that relaxes you and takes you out of your usual work/children/chores routine.

■ If you work a regular week, Sunday night is always the worst for sleep as your subconscious thoughts are full of the week ahead. Moreover, a relaxed weekend can mean that by Sunday night you are less tired and may find it harder to get to sleep. It helps to have a light, early evening dinner, and avoid alcohol or coffee on Sunday evenings.

Stress is ageing. Take time, especially as you get older, to replenish your energy.

■ Go for a massage, or ask your partner to give you a massage for 15 minutes or so and return the compliment.

■ An afternoon nap (calling it a siesta may make it sound more glamorous) is a great regenerator, allowing your body to digest lunch at the proper time and invigorating you for the afternoon.

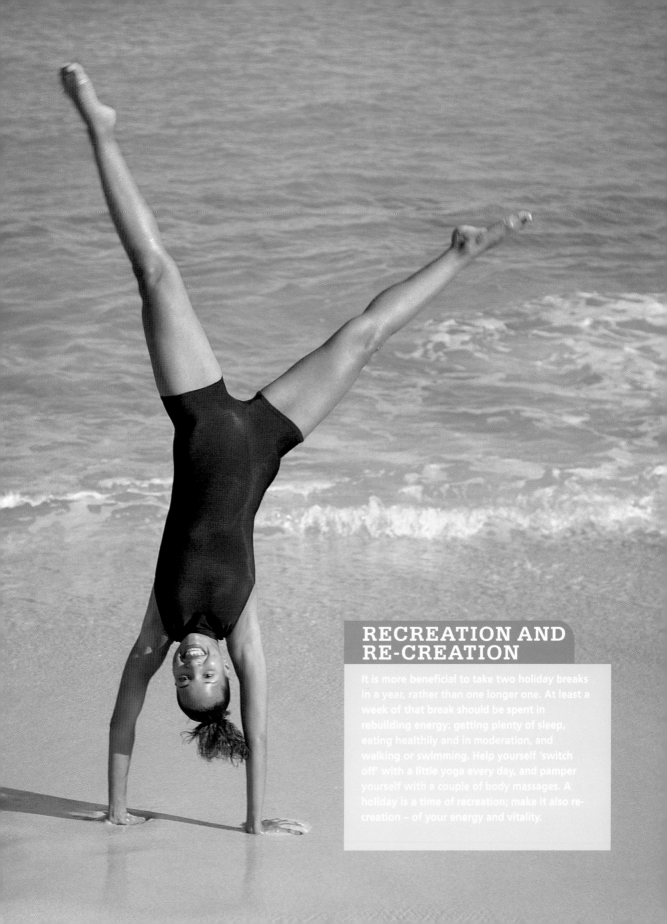

## RECREATION AND RE-CREATION

It is more beneficial to take two holiday breaks in a year, rather than one longer one. At least a week of that break should be spent in rebuilding energy: getting plenty of sleep, eating healthily and in moderation, and walking or swimming. Help yourself 'switch off' with a little yoga every day, and pamper yourself with a couple of body massages. A holiday is a time of recreation; make it also re-creation – of your energy and vitality.

# Defusing stress

Whenever you get stressed and angry, divert your mind to help the physical tension evaporate.

- Re-read a favourite book or watch a comedy or escapist romantic film on TV.

- There are many recordings available of sounds of nature. Choose something that is soothing but not monotonous, so that it keeps your focus of attention. Music, especially something classical or easy to listen to, has a similarly calming effect.

- Indulge in some happy visualization. Perhaps remember a moment in your life when you were overawed by nature – lakes mirroring snow-clad mountains, sunset over the sea, a misty valley at dawn. Let the image, colour and sounds reverberate in your mind.

## ULTIMATE CONTROL

I have witnessed yogis performing extraordinary feats that go beyond walking on hot charcoal or lying on a bed of nails. Once, a yogi was buried for a week, while scientists monitored his bodily functions electronically. In effect, he went into hibernation, breathing occasionally and his heart beating only rarely. One of the sadhus I would frequently visit in the Himalayas actually underwent samadhi, dying at will, three days before I arrived. He had warned his family and, on the designated day, called them to sit beside him. He told them that he was going to sleep after breakfast and asked not to be disturbed. After an hour he was dead.

# Controlling involuntary reactions

While some of our bodily functions are controlled at will, others are involuntary. The cortex, or outer surface, of the brain controls voluntary functions and is also responsible for such processes as analysis, decision-making and reasoning. The involuntary, or autonomous, nervous system controls everything else: digestion, heartbeat, hormone secretion, breathing and so on.

It is possible, however, to exercise some control over these involuntary functions. We can all interrupt the normal working of our lungs, for instance, by holding our breath. But with practice and by evolving meditative powers, this control can be taken much further. One of my yoga masters, Swami Ram Lakhan, can slow his pulse from his normal 62 beats per minute to 40 beats per minute.

Of all the subconscious functions of the body, breathing is the one most easily controlled at will. Controlled breathing and associated meditation are excellent and very effective methods of warding off stress. As well as relaxing physical tension, they:

- help you clear your mind of clutter and enable you to think more cogently

- give you a better appreciation of priorities

- recharge your batteries

- help you retain a good balance between different aspects of your life.

The Lifestyle Programme describes how to achieve slow, controlled breathing, using your lungs to the full (page 73) and then how to focus on the relaxation of different parts of the body in turn (page 74). The whole aim is to calm the mind and body, keeping your focus constant without falling asleep. See also Regaining Control, page 256.

# Anxiety and depression
Unlike most of the disorders described in this book, problems such as depression and eating disorders are seldom recognized in oneself, so this section is addressed to parents, partners and others closely involved in the lives of a sufferer.

The two principal psychological reactions to long-term stress are anxiety and depression. To a certain extent, these are the opposites of each other – manic-depression is also called bi-polar disorder. Put very basically, we either become manic (hyperactive, unable to relax, a 'bundle of nerves') or depressive (inert, lacking in energy and sluggish in thought).

## A ROYAL CURE

Avicenna, the great physician of the tenth century, was once asked to see the ruler of a princely state in central Asia. The prince couldn't walk, and was depressed and weak. Avicenna examined him thoroughly. Then he summoned the court and all the prince's ministers and aides. In their presence, Avicenna stood in front of the prince and began to insult him with strong, abusive language. To make matters worse, he cursed him and ran out of the palace. The ruler was so furious that he ran after the physician. There was pandemonium. Avicenna was punished heavily but, as he pointed out, he had cured the prince of his walking difficulties and depression.

## Helping depression

Curing depression is obviously not a matter of inducing anger or anxiety – that's simply substituting one disabling condition for another, and although the inertia and lethargy are temporarily ousted, the depression is still there. But a rush of one emotion does block another, and as depression feeds off itself, anything that replaces it, even for a short time, makes a positive contribution. Some yoga postures encourage you to laugh out loud when you are depressed, sad or grieving, or simply to cry to release blocked emotions.

Effective counters to depression are what a depressed person lacks, yet resists: exercise and a feeling of joy.

Exercise of any type helps improve the circulation of blood and releases compounds in the brain that have a beneficial effect on mood. It is characteristic that a depressive person is going to find it difficult to recognize the problem and be reluctant to accept help, but do all you can to encourage outdoor activities that increase oxygen supply and even overcome resistance to physical exercise. (Exertion should not be overdone, as fatigue is an element of depression, so sufficient rest is also important.)

Serotonin is a compound in the brain that plays a major role in mood control. Low levels of it induce depression but euphoria releases it in greater amounts – happiness begets happiness. Being in relaxed, happy company, watching a funny film or play, sharing jokes, all have a positive effect: laughter really is good medicine. What induces euphoria or tickles the funny bone is a very individual thing, so if you are helping a depressed person you may need to choose carefully – the excited laughter of exuberant children having fun may be magically contagious to one person but irritating to another.

*Other steps that can help:*

◆ neck massage, to improve blood flow to the brain
◆ general massage, to bring a pleasant sense of relaxation rather than a dragging feeling of inertia
◆ consulting a qualified homeopath or medical herbalist (St John's wort is often effective, but needs careful prescribing)
◆ allowing as much natural light into your home as possible.

See also Aids for Both Depression and Anxiety, below.

# Helping anxiety

Anxiety often manifests itself in hyperactivity and hypertension, so measures to counteract these reactions are helpful.

■ Avoid foods and drinks that contribute to a 'hyper' feeling: coffee, salt, alcohol, excess protein, very spicy food and, of course, recreational drugs that act as 'uppers'.

■ Eat more 'cooling' foods: cucumber, yoghurt, melon, parsley, squash, spinach, okra, fish, buttermilk, and calming herbal teas such as peppermint and chamomile.

Have a whole-body therapeutic massage regularly. The touch, the soothing effect of stimulating the skin and improved blood flow to the brain all have a calming influence. Tensed muscles relax, circulation improves and the heart rate slows down. You can massage your body yourself, focusing on the head, neck, jaw, calves, the palms of your hands and the soles of your feet. Anger tightens the jaw, so massaging it is an aid to relaxation.

# Aids for both depression and anxiety

Therapy takes many forms, and a professional will be able to bring an empathetic but dispassionate mind to the problem. Some people respond better one-to-one, while others find group therapy helpful, sharing thoughts and experiences and seeing that others have similar difficulties. (In extended families where the members are close-knit and share their thoughts and problems, there are fewer incidents of depression and psychological problems.)

■ Relaxation tapes or CDs, or relaxation classes, will help mind and body to relax. The techniques will induce better sleep, an important factor for all forms of anxiety and depression. A good night's sleep is revitalizing.

■ Yoga, especially yogic breathing (see pages 73–4), is beneficial in restoring balance and peace to the mind as well as the body.

■ Setting time aside for contemplation and meditation, to help harness thoughts and regulate emotions, is invaluable. It takes a bit of training and practice and it is easy to plead there is no time, but resolving emotional problems is something that should be regarded as a priority.

## MEDITATION

An instructor or mentor is a great help in the basics of meditation, but you may find you are able to enter a meditative state without help. Try the following:

■ Find somewhere quiet where you will not be disturbed either by other people or distracting surroundings.

■ If possible sit in the lotus position, on the floor, or upright on a cushion. Alternatively you could lie down or even sit on a chair. There should be no strain on your body and you should be comfortable without collapsing completely.

■ Use something to focus your thoughts, such as a candle flame or an imaginary spot on your forehead. Keep your body relaxed but still, so there is no movement to cause any 'ripples' in the mind. Let your body feel liberated of all tension, pain and discomfort.

It may not come at first, but with practice you'll develop an ability to enter a free-floating state in which your mind is freed from the clutches of the body and you achieve a definite sense of freedom and exhilaration. For more on meditation techniques and styles, see Regaining Control by Letting Go, overleaf.

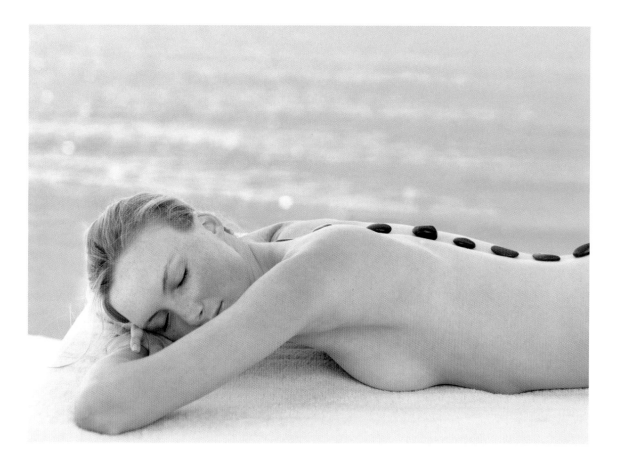

# Regaining control by letting go

In Indian tradition, various ways of regulating your mind use different instruments (tra) as a medium.

■ Yantra uses an object (yan = apparatus) to help focus or clear the mind. Prayer beads, a prayer wheel, a picture or statue are all popular methods; Indian sadhus use a metal fork-like device, a pincet, with numerous rings around it.

■ Mantra uses the mind (man) as the enabling instrument. Methods include:

◆ chanting (japa): repeating the same word or phrase ('Ohm' is probably the best known) until it reverberates in the mind and helps to calm the brain waves.
◆ concentration (dhyana): focusing on the forehead, as if looking at the moon, the sun or a coloured spot. This helps to drive out unwanted or disturbing thoughts.

With complete mastery over concentration (tapah), you can learn to lift your thoughts beyond your mind as if to unite with a universal force. A still, peaceful and highly controlled mind begins to reach levels of para-consciousness or trance. You may have out-of-body experiences where you feel detached from your physical body. It is in this state that, with much practice, you can develop control over bodily functions.

■ Tantra uses the body itself (tan) as the instrument, through controlled breathing and movements, meditation, simple diet and sublimation. Since reaching this peak of control and release of self is a feeling similar to that of orgasm, tantra has gained connotations with sexual sublimity (see the chapter on Sexual Health, page 124). As the matter of sex always remained a taboo among practitioners, it was not openly taught or discussed and tantra became a rare and mystified subject. There are probably only a select few who are true masters of tantra.